Sexual Dysfunction

Sexual Dysfunction

A Guide for Assessment and Treatment

SECOND EDITION

JOHN P. WINCZE

MICHAEL P. CAREY

Series Editor's Note by David H. Barlow

Foreword by Sandra R. Leiblum

THE GUILFORD PRESS
New York London

© 2001 The Guilford Press
A Division of Guilford Publications, Inc.
72 Spring Street, New York, NY 10012
www.guilford.com

Printed in the United States of America

This book is printed on acid-free paper.

Last digit is print number: 9   8   7   6   5   4   3   2   1

Library of Congress Cataloging-in-Publication Data

Wincze, John P., 1943–
    Sexual dysfunction: a guide for assessment and treatment / John P. Wincze,
Michael P. Carey; series editor's note by David H. Barlow; foreword by
Sandra R. Lieblum.—2nd ed.
      p. ; cm.—(Treatment manuals for practitioners)
Includes bibliographical references and index.
ISBN 1-57230-540-1 (pbk.: alk. paper)
    1. Sexual disorders—Diagnosis—Handbooks, manuals, etc.   2. Sexual
disorders—Treatment—Handbooks, manuals, etc.   I. Carey, Michael P.
II. Title.   III. Series.
    [DNLM: 1. Sexual Dysfunctions, Psychological—diagnosis.   2. Sexual
Dysfunctions, Psychological—therapy.   WM 611 W758s 2001]
RC556 .W564 2001
616.85′83—dc21

                                        2001023866

About the Authors

John P. Wincze, a licensed clinical psychologist, is currently Clinical Professor of Psychology in the Department of Psychology at Brown University and Adjunct Professor of Psychology in the Department of Psychology at Boston University. He received his BA from Wesleyan University, his MA from Boston College, and his PhD from the University of Vermont. Dr. Wincze currently serves as an Associate Editor of the *Journal of Sex Research*. He has published more than 100 articles and chapters in the areas of sexual dysfunction and deviations.

Michael P. Carey, a licensed clinical psychologist, is Director of the Center for Health and Behavior and Professor of Psychology at Syracuse University. He received his BA from St. Lawrence University and his MA and PhD from Vanderbilt University. Dr. Carey has served on the editorial boards of the *Journal of Consulting and Clinical Psychology, Health Psychology, Psychological Assessment, Archives of Sexual Behavior,* and *Clinical Psychology Review.* He has published 150 articles and chapters in the areas of sexual health, health promotion, and coping with chronic illness.

Acknowledgments

We wish to thank many individuals for their contributions to the writing of this book. Special thanks to Michele Barchi, Teal Pedlow, Mary Beth Pray, and Markus Wiegel for their technical assistance with the preparation and proofing of the manuscript. We would like to extend our gratitude to David Barlow for his invitation to contribute to this fine series, and to Sandra Leiblum for her generous foreword. A special thank you to Barbara Watkins of The Guilford Press for her many helpful suggestions to improve our work. The work of Michael Carey was made possible by an Independent Scientist Award from the National Institute of Mental Health.

We would like to dedicate this book to several special people. John would like to dedicate his efforts to the enduring and privileged friendships of Lee and Barbara, Bob and Linda, and Dick and Diane. Your support, humor, and love have provided inspiration and meaning through celebrations and challenging times. John would also like to dedicate his efforts to Benjamin, Henry, and J. Harrison, who have added new dimensions to love and to the purpose of life.

Michael would like to dedicate his efforts to his family, especially his late mother, Alice, who gave more than one lifetime's worth of love, vitality, and kindness to us all; to his father, Jerry, and his sister, Debbie, for their courage and caregiving; to Ed and Katie, for their compassion and commitment to family; and to Alison and Maureen, for making the sun rise and the stars twinkle.

Series Editor's Note

Since the appearance of direct behavioral approaches to sexual dysfunctions made popular by Masters and Johnson, the impression has grown that there is little more to learn about treating the variety of common sexual problems that patients so often present to health care professionals. Nothing could be further from the truth. Early reports of success with specific sexual dysfunctions proved tantalizingly difficult to reproduce in the offices of numerous clinicians around the country. With this development, the fad of doing sex therapy passed and it is now very hard to find a competent, knowledgeable sex therapist outside of our major cities. Furthermore, there has been a veritable explosion of information in the area of sexual function and dysfunction, much of it coming from our medical colleagues. New procedures and techniques emanating from various medical specialities have resulted in advances that are being widely utilized in the care and management of sexual dysfunction, with the initial success of Viagra for erectile dysfunction the most visible. But it has also become clear, even with erectile dysfunction, that only approximately one-third of patients are satisfied with the results of pharmacotherapy alone (Virag, 1999).

Now, John Wincze and Michael Carey, two of the most experienced sex researchers and therapists in the United States, have revised an important guide for therapists who wish to be knowledgeable about and utilize the latest procedures for treating sexual dysfunctions. Clinicians reading this book will benefit from the authors' long years of clinical experience with a variety of sexual dysfunctions, and will also become conversant with the latest procedures from both medicine and psychology in use today. Awareness of the effects of such new approaches as Viagra, vasoactive therapy, and related strategies will prove valuable to those confronting sexual problems. As the authors point out, clinicians with relatively little experience should be able to use these programs to treat the majority of sexual dysfunctions with which they are confronted and be confident that their approaches are based on the latest developments in our science.

DAVID H. BARLOW

Foreword

It is refreshing to find a book that truly delivers what it promises. Wincze and Carey's second edition of *Sexual Dysfunction: A Guide to Assessment and Treatment* does just that. It provides a timely, sensible and practical approach to evaluating and treating the major sexual dysfunctions and it does so in a no-nonsense, straightforward, and readable way.

Today, more than ever, individuals and couples want to enjoy sex. With sexual images and allusions bombarding us from all sides and promises of quick fixes for sexual problems crowding the pages of popular magazines and newspapers, it is not surprising that most people want and expect sexual satisfaction. Yet there are few reliable resources for individuals experiencing sexual difficulties. Physicians often avoid asking patients about their sexual concerns, let alone having (or taking) the time to counsel patients. Even when they are comfortable about initiating sexual inquiry, medical doctors tend to over-emphasize the biological basis of problems and neglect the psychological and interpersonal determinants of difficulties. The internet, on the other hand, is full of sex-related sites and materials, but few can be trusted to reliably or accurately provide genuine guidance for overcoming sexual difficulties. If it is erotic stimulation or access to sexual partners that is sought, the internet delivers. But if treatment is what is called for, most individuals would be better served by consulting a skilled therapist. Unfortunately, most clinicians, while well intentioned and sympathetic, are unaware of the latest and most effective approaches to the assessment and treatment of sexual dysfunction.

This is why this book is so valuable. It not only provides a scholarly overview of the major male and female sexual dysfunctions, it reminds the reader that the etiology of most sexual difficulties is over determined—that predisposing, precipitating, and maintaining factors of both a physical and psychological nature are often sexual culprits. The authors write from a well-reasoned and researched cognitive-behavioral approach—one that clinicians of any orientation can find helpful.

Each chapter includes sections updating the prevalence, etiology, and multiple biological and psychosocial contributions to the dysfunction under discussion and offers both psychological and pharmacological approaches to treatment. The authors provide clinical vignettes illustrating their recommendations, but more importantly, include the actual assessment instruments and questionnaires, interview outlines, and referral and follow-up letters that enhance clinical practice. It is hard to imagine that any reader—whether novice or expert—will come away from this volume without having learned something useful.

Wincze and Carey are to be congratulated for offering a succinct, scholarly, and above all sane approach to the assessment and treatment of sexual difficulties. They deliver what they promise.

SANDRA R. LEIBLUM, PHD
Director, Center for Sexual and Marital Health
Robert Wood Johnson Medical School
Piscataway, New Jersey

Contents

Sexual Dysfunction

1

Overview of This Book

Interest in sexual behavior increased dramatically in the last two decades. During the 1980s (and continuing to the present), the emergence of HIV and AIDS raised awareness of the health implications of sexual behavior. During the 1990s, there have been highly visible developments in the pharmacological treatment of sexual problems, most notably, the development and marketing of Viagra (sildenafil citrate) for the treatment of erectile dysfunction. Private and publicly supported research promises more pharmacological treatments of sexual problems in the decade to come.

With the launching of Viagra and subsequent worldwide attention, questions were raised about the need for psychological treatments. Doubts about the role of mental health professionals in treating sex dysfunction have been short-lived. Although Viagra alone as treatment has been sufficient for some men suffering from erectile dysfunction, for many others this has not been the case. Viagra has not cured marital and relationship problems, has not corrected myths and misunderstandings (nor has it provided accurate educational material), has not overridden negative sexual messages and sexual trauma, and has not taught sexual skills (nor how best to create sexual feelings and a conducive sexual environment). No pharmacological agent will substitute for these basic and essential ingredients of enjoyable and fulfilling sexual experiences.

Viagra has had the most impact on primary care physicians, who are the largest prescribers of this medication. Unfortunately, primary care physicians do not typically have the time or skills to screen sexual problems adequately and often prescribe Viagra when nonmedical factors may be contributing heavily to the problem. Viagra "failures" are most likely a result of insufficient psychosocial screening and a purely biomedical approach to a complex, bio-psychosocial experience.

A decided benefit of the Viagra craze is that it has legitimized help seeking for sexual problems. With the frequent commercial appearances of former U.S. senator and presidential hopeful Bob Dole (extolling the benefits of Viagra for treating erectile dysfunction), the American public has been given a very powerful message that sexual problems are commonplace *and* treatable, and there is no need for shame.

Sex is important to people. This is more evident today than at any other time in our history. Our goals in writing this book are (1) to provide a state-of-the-science overview of the most common sexual dysfunctions, and (2) to present an introductory guide to the assessment and treatment of these problems.

This book is intended for health care professionals at various levels of expertise and for both medical and nonmedical disciplines. Accomplished sex therapists may wish to compare their own approaches with ours and may find some interesting ideas described herein. This book is also intended for health care professionals currently in training (e.g., graduate students, medical interns, and residents), or currently practicing but who have little (or no) previous training in the assessment and treatment of sexual dysfunctions. Finally, this book is also intended for practicing physicians (e.g., internists, family practitioners, urologists, and gynecologists) who treat patients' sexual dysfunction complaints and who wish to learn more about the psychological aspects of sexual dysfunction. This book is not intended to replace other types of formal training and should be used in conjunction with supervision from an experienced sex therapist.

We begin in this chapter with an overview of our current understanding of sexual function and dysfunction, and describe our general approach to the management of sexual difficulties. The remainder of the book is divided into two parts and incorporates the most up-to-date clinical and research information available. In Part I (Chapters 2–5), we provide a more detailed discussion of each of the main classes of sexual dysfunction. We focus on definitions and descriptions, prevalence, and etiology. In Part II (Chapters 6–10), we describe our approach to assessing and treating these problems, present seven detailed case histories, and provide information about how you can obtain further training and even establish a practice in sex therapy.

Definitions of Sexual Function and Dysfunction

Controversy and Change

We are educators, clinicians, and researchers. In the context of our teaching and supervision, we often wrestle with the constructs of "normality and abnormality," "health and pathology," and "function and dysfunction." We are thankful that our students and supervisees continually challenge our definitions and help us to remain open-minded and responsive to new information. This is particularly important in a socially sensitive and value-laden field such as human sexuality—a field where popular beliefs about function and dysfunction seem to be quite labile. To illustrate this point, we can use two examples: thinking about masturbation and sexual desire.

In previous times, masturbation received widespread condemnation. For example, in the 18th century, numerous treatises were written describing the physical and mental consequences of masturbation (see Caird & Wincze, 1977; Gagnon, 1977). It was during this time that a particularly well-known Swiss physician, Tissot (1766), published a volume titled *Onania, or a Treatise upon the Disorders Produced by Masturbation*. Among the many physical and mental disorders purportedly caused by masturbation were failing eyesight, consumption, gonorrhea, hemorrhoids, digestive disorders, melancholy, catalepsy, imbecility, loss of sensation, lethargy, pervasive weakness of the nervous system, impotence, and insanity! Eventually, because of the scientific work of Kinsey and others, more enlightened views about masturbation emerged. Today, in stark contrast, masturbation is prescribed as therapy (e.g., see LoPiccolo & Lobitz, 1972; Zilbergeld, 1999). In fact, it turns out that directed masturbation (see Chapter 7) is a particularly effective treatment for lifelong female orgasmic disorder (see Heiman & LoPiccolo, 1988). (As an aside, we are reminded of the exchange between the Countess and Boris in Woody Allen's movie *Love and Death*. Countess: "You are a wonderful lover." Boris: "I practice a lot when I am alone.")

Before we rest on our accomplishments, however, we should note that we are not entirely free of 18th-century thinking. It was just a few years ago that Surgeon General Jocelyn Elders was forced to resign her post for suggesting that masturbation might be an acceptable substitute for high-risk sexual behavior! Yes, change has occurred, but there is still room for improvement.

Related beliefs about sexual appetite, desire, and behavior have also changed. Beginning with the writing of the Christian theologian Paul, sexual abstinence and chastity were seen as virtuous. Indeed, those interested in maximizing their spiritual development were required to take vows of celibacy and chastity (Cole, 1956). In the first half of the 20th century, however, scientists began to question whether sexual abstinence was contrary to human beings' basic biological nature (e.g., Parshley, 1933) and potentially harmful. Today, the absence of sexual desire is seen as a clinical disorder that warrants proper diagnosis and treatment. Who knows what the next decade will bring?

We hope that these two examples (from many that we might have selected) serve to illustrate our point: Definitions of sexual function and dysfunction are inevitably influenced by current social mores, values, and knowledge. In the past 10 years, we have noticed an increase in sexual dysfunction research studies from different cultures. Whenever possible, we have incorporated cross-cultural comparisons. As these and other influences change, so too will our definitions of sexual function and dysfunction. Mindful of this caveat, then, we are poised to discuss current clinical definitions.

Current Definitions

Current approaches to define sexual function and dysfunction have been influenced by recent biomedical research and clinical practice. Current thinking suggests that human sexual functioning, for most people on most occasions, proceeds sequentially. This axiom, accepted by most sexologists (i.e., experts in human sexuality), has its formal beginning with Havelock Ellis (1906), who postulated that sexual functioning has two stages: tumescence (i.e., the engorgement of genitals with blood, resulting in erection in males and vaginal lubrication in females) and detumescence (i.e., the outflow of blood from the genitals following orgasm). Ever since, scientist–practitioners have attempted to delineate more precisely the basic biological sequencing of sexual function.

William Masters and Virginia Johnson, household names to most Americans, contributed immensely to our understanding of sexual functioning. During the 1950s and 1960s, they conducted a very extensive (and equally controversial) series of scientific observations of sexual activity with human volunteers. In their 1966 book *Human Sexual Response*, based upon thousands of hours of careful laboratory research, Masters and Johnson suggested that physiological responding in healthy, well-functioning adults proceeds through four stages: (1) excitement, (2) plateau, (3) orgasm, and (4) resolution. They documented the genital and extragenital physiological changes that typically occur during each of these phases. The model they provided was instructive and elegant.

Yet something was missing. That something was most apparent to those practitioners working with not-so-well-functioning individuals and couples (e.g., Kaplan, 1979; Lief, 1977). Some of these sexually troubled persons complained of an inability to become amorous, a lack of interest in sex, or even an aversion to sexual activity. In the decade following the publication of *Human Sexual Response*, it became increasingly clear that there was a "stage" preliminary to the excitement phase identified and described by Masters and Johnson. This preliminary stage, subsequently labeled sexual "desire," involved a person's cognitive and affective readiness for, and interest in, sexual activity. Without sexual desire, physiological and subjective arousal, and subsequent orgasm were much less likely to occur.

Subsequent theoretical writing and empirical research have served as the basis for our current understanding of sexual function and dysfunction. Most sexologists agree that healthy sexual functioning comprises three primary stages: desire, arousal, and orgasm. (Each of these terms is defined and discussed further in the coming chapters.) Sexual dysfunction, then, consists of an impairment or disturbance in one of these stages. Although this stage model is somewhat arbitrary in that it identifies discrete stages in what may well be a continuous process, we believe that it provides a useful heuristic from which to conceptualize and discuss sexual health. Not surprisingly, this model is compatible with current diagnostic schemes.

Recognizing Sexual Dysfunctions: The Challenge of Diagnosis

The Current Diagnostic Scheme

Although several diagnostic approaches have been proposed to classify the sexual dysfunctions (e.g., Schover, Friedman, Weiler, Heiman, & LoPiccolo, 1982), the diagnostic scheme that has been most widely adopted for sexual dysfunctions is that contained in the *Diagnostic and Statistical Manual of Mental Disorders* (hereafter abbreviated as DSM; American Psychiatric Association, 1994). This series of manuals was developed to aid mental health care professionals in the diagnosis and treatment of the so-called "mental disorders." (The first edition of DSM appeared in 1952, and new editions appeared in 1968 and 1980; the third edition was revised in 1987. The fourth edition of DSM was published in 1994 and its text revision—DSM-IV-TR—in 2000.) Although the manual was not developed for sex therapists, it contains diagnostic categories and criteria for the most commonly seen sexual difficulties.

There are nine major diagnostic categories for sexual dysfunction in DSM-IV-TR. These diagnostic categories, depicted in Table 1.1, include the following: hypoactive sexual desire disorder, sexual aversion disorder, female

TABLE 1.1. Categories of Sexual Dysfunction among Men and Women

Phase of response cycle affected	Men	Women
Desire	Hypoactive sexual desire disorder	Hypoactive sexual desire disorder
	Sexual aversion disorder	Sexual aversion disorder
Arousal	Male erectile disorder	Female sexual arousal disorder
Orgasm	Male orgasmic disorder	Female orgasmic disorder
	Premature ejaculation	
Pain	Dyspareunia	Dyspareunia
		Vaginismus

sexual arousal disorder, male erectile disorder, female orgasmic disorder, male orgasmic disorder, premature ejaculation, dyspareunia, and vaginismus. (These terms, and their diagnostic criteria, are described in detail in Chapters 2–5.) All nine of the dysfunctions identified in DSM-IV-TR should be further conceptualized along two dimensions. First, they may be characterized as "lifelong" (also known as "primary") or "acquired" (also known as "secondary"). Second, a dysfunction may be "generalized" (i.e., occurring across all sexual situations and partners) or "situational" (i.e., limited to certain situations and partners). These distinctions are believed to be important with respect to both etiology and treatment.

DSM-IV-TR represented an improvement over previous editions of DSM but is still far from perfect. The primary limitations within sexual dysfunction diagnosis is the inherent subjectivity of criteria in most categories. Terms such as "minimal sexual stimulation" or "normal sexual excitement" leave much to clinical judgment.

Despite limitations, DSM-IV-TR classifications continue to be used in professional journal articles, by most health professionals (from whom referrals may originate), and by insurance companies (for third-party reimbursement). It should be noted, however, that most insurance companies still do not reimburse for treatment of sexual dysfunction. Often, a diagnosis of anxiety disorder or depression is justifiable. Familiarity with DSM-IV-TR categories and criteria is essential.

Sexual Deviations, Dysfunctions, and Dissatisfaction

The DSM diagnostic scheme includes the sexual deviations (i.e., paraphilias), as well as sexual dysfunctions. Paraphilias are disorders in which an individual experiences recurrent and intense sexual urges and fantasies involving either (1) nonhuman objects (i.e., a fetish), (2) suffering or humiliation of oneself or one's partner (i.e., sadomasochism), or (3) nonconsenting partners (e.g., pedophilia, exhibitionism, frotteurism). Assessment and treatment of the paraphilias are not covered in this book. (Interested readers are referred to Kafka, 2000; Laws, 1989; Laws & O'Donohue, 1997; Wincze, 2000.)

However, knowledge of the assessment and treatment of the paraphilias or atypical sexual behavior (that does not meet the criteria for paraphilia) is important for assessment and treatment of sexual dysfunction. Unusual types of sexual preferences or stimulation are at times at the root of sexual dysfunction in both men and women. Incorporating or controlling the atypical sexual behavior of one partner within a couple's sexual practices may be an important component of the treatment of sexual dysfunction. Therapists treating sexual dysfunction problems can best serve their patients by being knowledgeable of and comfortable with "atypical" sexual behaviors.

In addition to being willing to explore, understand, and accept a person's unusual sexual practices and preferences, the therapist dealing with sexual dysfunction problems must also understand and accept that not everyone is concerned or distressed by their sexual dysfunction. Indeed, DSM-IV-TR includes the criteria of distress and/or interpersonal difficulty for each sexual dysfunction description (i.e., "The disturbance causes marked distress or interpersonal difficulty").

Thus, a person may be "dysfunctional" but not necessarily dissatisfied. In a landmark study published in the *New England Journal of Medicine*, Frank, Anderson, and Rubenstein (1978) investigated 100 happily married American couples. These researchers attempted to determine the frequency of sexual dysfunctions experienced and the relationship of these problems to sexual satisfaction. Although over 80% of the couples reported that their marital and sexual relations were happy and satisfying, 40% of the men reported erectile and ejaculatory dysfunction, and 63% of the women reported arousal or orgasmic dysfunction! Even more surprising was the finding that the number of dysfunctions was *not* strongly associated with overall sexual satisfaction. These findings have been corroborated in a similar study conducted by Nettelbladt and Uddenberg (1979) in Europe. These authors reported that sexual dysfunction was *not* significantly related to sexual satisfaction in their sample of 58 married Swedish men.

These empirical findings remind us that sexual health involves more than just intact physiology and typical "functioning" (i.e., progression through desire, arousal, and orgasm phases). In our culture, and in many others as well, sexual health is enhanced to the extent that it occurs in a rich interpersonal context that involves respect and trust, open lines of communication, and mutual commitment to all aspects of the relationship. (This is not to say that other approaches to sexual behavior are wrong, but rather to describe the conditions under which sexual satisfaction is maximized.) Sexual health is most likely to occur in individuals who are psychologically as well as neurologically, hormonally, and vascularly intact. Because existing diagnostic schemas, which focus exclusively on sexual "functioning," cannot encompass the richness of sexual health, such schemas (and diagnoses in general) have been criticized (e.g., Schover et al., 1982; Szasz, 1980; Wincze, 1982). This limitation notwithstanding, most scientist–practitioners find the DSM classification schema useful for communicating among themselves, for presenting information about subclasses of problems, and for treatment planning. Indeed, the existence of the diagnostic system allows researchers to conduct epidemiological studies in order to determine the frequency with which disorders occur.

Prevalence of the Sexual Dysfunctions

With the recent explosion of interest in sexual dysfunction due to pharmacological treatments, there is every reason to believe that sexual dysfunctions are prevalent psychological disorders in the general population. Simons and

Carey (2001) point out that although sexual disorders tend *not* to be included in large-scale epidemiological studies, there have been 52 empirical studies since 1990 that provide data on sexual dysfunctions. Comparing various prevalence rates across studies can be misleading, however, because studies differ in research methodology, definition of sexual disorders, and the sample under study (e.g., a sample drawn from a diabetes clinic cannot be compared to one drawn at random from a community). Nonetheless, we now have some confidence in the prevalence range for most sexual dysfunctions within the general population. Community samples indicate a current prevalence ranging up to 3% for male orgasmic disorder, 5% for erectile disorder, 3% for male hypoactive sexual desire disorder, 10% for female orgasmic disorder and 5% for premature ejaculation (Simons & Carey, 2001). These prevalence data are consistent with anecdotal evidence from practicing social workers, psychologists, psychiatrists, and primary care nurses and physicians whose patients complain frequently about sexual dysfunction problems.

Etiology of the Sexual Dysfunctions

To treat sexual dysfunction or dissatisfaction effectively, it is helpful (but probably not necessary) to understand how that dysfunction or dissatisfaction developed. Unfortunately, our understanding of the cause(s) of the sexual dysfunctions remains incomplete. Moreover, much of our understanding comes from clinical observation rather than well-controlled research. As in the study of disease and psychopathology, this is not unusual; however, we do need to be mindful of the methodological limitations of such quasi-experimental research, cautious about our judgments, and continually open to new clinical and research data.

 With these caveats in mind, we are nonetheless confident about the following general statements regarding the etiology of the sexual dysfunctions:

 1. In most cases, sexual difficulties are multiply determined; that is, there is usually not just a single cause for a problem; rather, one can expect to find an array of factors that contribute to the development of a sexual difficulty. Appreciation of this principle can help to explain why treatments need to be customized to the individual, as well as why treatments need to be empirically eclectic, multimodal (Lazarus, 1988), or broad-spectrum (LoPiccolo & Friedman, 1988) rather than dogmatically designed and narrowly focused.

 2. Within such a multicausal context, causes can be organized for communication purposes into three temporal categories (Hawton, 1985). First, "predisposing" factors are those prior life experiences (e.g., childhood sexual trauma) and inherited characteristics (e.g., diabetes) that make a person vulnerable to certain types of dysfunction. These predisposing factors serve

as diatheses that place an individual at risk; predisposing factors may be necessary, but they are rarely sufficient to produce a dysfunction. Second, "precipitating" (or triggering) factors (e.g., stress associated with job difficulties) are those life events and experiences associated with the initial onset of a symptom or dysfunction. A precipitating factor serves as the proverbial "straw that broke the camel's back." Third, "maintaining" factors (e.g., lack of privacy) are those ongoing life circumstances or physical conditions that help to explain why a dysfunction persists.

3. Causes can also be classified, again for heuristic purposes, into three human systems or frames of reference. First, causes may be inherently biological or medical. Thus, for example, the presence of penile microangiopathy (i.e., small-vessel disease) in a middle-aged male diabetic can cause erectile difficulties. Similarly, the hormonal changes that can accompany menopause in women can produce vaginal dryness and dyspareunia. Second, causes can be psychological in nature. Gross disturbances in reality testing (e.g., paranoid delusions), major depression, and serious anxiety disorders have all been implicated in the pathogenesis of sexual dysfunction. Less obvious psychological contributions to dysfunction include negative body image and fear of negative evaluation or rejection. Finally, causes can arise from a person's social context. At the dyadic level, factors such as poor communication and relationship inequalities can foster sexual dysfunction. Larger sociocultural influences, such as sex-role or religious proscriptions, may also have an impact upon sexual functioning.

In summary, we propose that the etiology of most sexual dysfunctions will be multiply determined, involving the transaction of biological, psychological, and social factors over a period of time. Thus, a major challenge for us as sex therapists is to recognize these multiple sources of influence, and to appreciate that sexual dysfunction represents but one manifestation of a complex process. As our knowledge of etiology increases, it is likely that we will also develop more reliable and valid assessments, as well as more efficacious treatments.

Assessment and Treatment

After introducing the dysfunctions in Part I of this book, we devote Part II to the assessment and treatment of sexual dysfunction and dissatisfaction. This material commences in Chapter 6. Before then, however, we wish to make clear the beliefs that influence our approach to assessment and treatment.

First, we are strong advocates of the biopsychosocial approach to health care, which has received increased attention in the training of many health care professionals (see Engel, 1977). This model has important implications for both assessment and treatment that will become manifest throughout this book. Clearly, this model requires continuing efforts to stay abreast of developments—not only in one's own discipline but also in related disciplines.

Second, we are equally committed to the scientist–practitioner model of health care training and delivery. This model, espoused by the American Psychological Association as its primary training approach, has been much misunderstood, misapplied, and subsequently criticized. However, as we understand it, this model requires practicing clinicians (1) to stay abreast of recent scientific developments and, more importantly, (2) to adopt an empirical approach to their work. We discuss each of these "requirements" in turn.

It is important to stay current and remain informed of recent advances, controversies, and other developments in our field. Certainly, the arrival of effective pharmacological treatments for some sexual dysfunction problems is a prime example of this. All clinicians working with male erectile dysfunction must now be informed of the advantages and limitations of Viagra.

The recommendation that one adopt a scientific approach to one's work requires careful, ongoing assessment and critical self-evaluation (see Barlow, Hayes, & Nelson, 1984; Carey, Flasher, Maisto, & Turkat, 1984). We believe that a scientific approach is especially necessary in a controversial and understudied area such as human sexuality, because there is an increased probability of conjecture and subjective (or even distorted) information. Thus, the scientist–practitioner approach, which sensitizes one to the need to be critical of current "knowledge," is especially valuable in a field that is susceptible to potentially harmful information.

Third, we believe that a wide variety of sexual practices and orientations have been prematurely labeled as psychopathological, deviant, or abnormal. Therefore, with some obvious exceptions (e.g., coercive sexual practices with a nonconsenting partner), we try not to make value judgments regarding the "rightness" or "wrongness" of practices that are not universally approved in our culture (e.g., gay and bisexual practices). Instead, we call for continued research and study of these practices to increase our understanding of the richness and diversity of human sexual expression.

We have attempted to prepare a book that is equally applicable to male and female, as well as to gay and straight, concerns. At points where our coverage seems biased or one-sided, please understand that this was not our intention; such instances may reflect the state of current knowledge or our inability to express ourselves as well as we would have liked.

Finally, we would like to encourage all professionals to adhere closely to the ethical principles of their disciplines. Because our own professional training is in psychology, we follow the guidelines proffered by the American Psychological Association. Further information is available from the *Casebook on Ethical Principles of Psychologists* (American Psychological Association, 1987), or from the state licensing boards of the various professions.

Part I

THE SEXUAL DYSFUNCTIONS

Sexual difficulties can be divided into three broad categories: the sexual dysfunctions, the paraphilias, and the gender identity and dysphoria disturbances. In the first part of this book, we provide an introduction to all of the sexual dysfunctions. Specifically, in Chapter 2, we discuss sexual desire disorders; in Chapter 3, we overview the sexual arousal disorders; in Chapter 4, we introduce the orgasmic disorders; and, in Chapter 5, we discuss the sexual pain disorders. In each chapter, we provide basic descriptions and information about the most common clinical presentations for each dysfunction. We also provide information on the prevalence and etiology of the dysfunctions. We provide separate chapters for each phase of the sexual response cycle, and a separate chapter for the sexual pain disorders, for three reasons: (1) to enhance your understanding of these dysfunctions when they occur in simple forms; (2) to provide you with a theoretical structure; and (3) to facilitate subsequent communication. This introductory material sets the stage for our discussion of the assessment and treatment of the sexual dysfunctions in Part II of the book.

2

Sexual Desire Disorders

It is always important to agree on what we mean when we use certain terms. However, when it comes to sexual "desire," agreeing on a definition is challenging because sexual desire is a construct that seems to have different meanings for different people. To nonprofessionals, desire is synonymous with "horniness" or "lust" or "passion." To mental health professionals, desire refers to the endpoint of a complex interaction of biological (e.g., neuro-endocrine), psychological (e.g., cognitive and affective), social (e.g., relationship), and cultural (e.g., religious upbringing) forces. For our purposes here, we define "desire" as an interest in being sexual and in having sexual relations by oneself or with an appropriate (e.g., mutually consenting) partner. Consistent with the consensus in the field, we suggest that "healthy" individuals living in situations that are not highly stressful will experience sexual desire regularly; moreover, such individuals will take advantage of appropriate opportunities for sexual expression when they arise. In contrast, individuals who are persistently and recurrently uninterested in sexual expression, who report the absence of sexual fantasies altogether, and who are distressed by this, are said to be experiencing low sexual desire.

Two additional points warrant mention. First, although our focus is on low sexual desire, brief mention should be made of "abnormally" high sexual desire. Disorders involving excessive sexual desire have enjoyed many names, including "sexual addiction," "sexual compulsion," "nymphomania," "satyriasis," or "Don Juanism." There is little agreement on the usage of these terms. The term "sexual addiction," in particular, has been used to explain such varied practices as frequent masturbation, impersonal sex, emotional dependency, and extramarital affairs. The practice of engaging in "excessive" sexual behavior has received increased attention in the era of AIDS. Instances of excessive desire do occur commonly in the paraphilias but, as mentioned earlier, this type of sexual disorder is not the focus of this book. Interested readers are referred to Coleman (1987, 1990), Laws (1989), and Laws and O'Donohue (1997) for more information about the sexual paraphilias. Second, it is important not to confuse sexual desire (interest) with sexual behavior. Spector, Carey, and Steinberg (1996) argue that sexual behavior is a poor measure of desire because behavior can occur without desire, and sexual desire can occur without an expression of sexual behavior.

Description and Clinical Presentation

Desire disorders in men and women are among the most challenging sexual problems for clinicians to diagnose, assess, and treat. They are often associated with other sexual problems, mental disorders, and medical conditions. Thus, a complaint of low sexual desire may also be associated with a number of other conditions or circumstances, such as sexual aversion or trauma, a lack of attraction or love toward one's partner, homoerotic attractions within a heterosexual relationship, a disparity in desire within a couple's relationship, depression, or as a consequence of another sexual problem or medical condition. Thus, diagnosis becomes quite challenging.

DSM-IV identifies two types of low desire disorders: hypoactive sexual desire disorder (HSDD; see Table 2.1) and sexual aversion disorder (SAD; see Table 2.2). To distinguish between these, one focuses on the affect associated with the report of low desire.

A person may report low desire for sexual activity along with neutral affect; that is, the person's attitude regarding sex is that he or she can "take it or leave it." Such a person has neither positive nor negative feelings about sexual expression. It is unlikely that such a person would seek professional assistance, and it is questionable whether such a person should be diagnosed at all (see Tobias, 1975). In fact, according to the diagnostic criteria in DSM-IV, a diagnosis should not be made if there is no "marked distress or interpersonal difficulty" (see Criterion B in Table 2.1).

More commonly, a person with low sexual desire reports that he or she is also experiencing negative affective states, including distress, sadness, disappointment, frustration, or embarrassment about having reduced or absent desire. Such persons, who may seek out (or be forced to enter) treatment, may feel guilty and depressed because of their absence of sexual interest and urges. This negative affect may be the result of a discrepancy between a person and his or her partner (see the case illustration presented later in this chapter), or between the person's behavior and socially transmitted expectations about what is "normal." In such cases, the appropriate diagnosis may be HSDD.

TABLE 2.1. Diagnostic Criteria for Hypoactive Sexual Desire Disorder (302.71)

A. Persistently or recurrently deficient (or absent) sexual fantasies and desire for sexual activity. The judgment of deficiency or absence is made by the clinician, taking into account factors that affect sexual functioning, such as age and the context of the person's life.

B. The disturbance causes marked distress or interpersonal difficulty.

C. The sexual dysfunction is not better accounted for by another Axis I disorder (except another Sexual Dysfunction) and is not due exclusively to the direct physiological effects of a substance (e.g., a drug of abuse, a medication) or a general medical condition.

Specify type:
Lifelong Type
Acquired Type

Specify type:
Generalized Type
Situational Type

Specify:
Due to Psychological Factors
Due to Combined Factors

Note. From American Psychiatric Association (2000). Copyright 2000 by the American Psychiatric Association. Reprinted by permission.

TABLE 2.2. Diagnostic Criteria for Sexual Aversion Disorder (302.79)

A. Persistent or recurrent extreme aversion to, and avoidance of, all (or almost all) genital sexual contact with a sexual partner.

B. The disturbance causes marked distress or interpersonal difficulty.

C. The sexual dysfunction is not better accounted for by another Axis I disorder (except another Sexual Dysfunction).

Specify type:
Lifelong Type
Acquired Type

Specify type:
Generalized Type
Situational Type

Specify:
Due to Psychological Factors
Due to Combined Factors

Note. From American Psychiatric Association (2000). Copyright 2000 by the American Psychiatric Association. Reprinted by permission.

A third alternative can be seen in the person with low sexual desire who is fearful of, and wishes to avoid, sexual activity. When avoidance of sex is accompanied by an extreme aversion to genital sexual contact, SAD is the more accurate diagnosis. Although we believe that HSDD and SAD are more accurately viewed as points along the same continuum, they have been conceptualized as qualitatively distinct diagnostic entities in DSM-IV-TR. In this view, SAD is characterized by fear and avoidance, whereas HSDD is typified by depression and a lack of response initiative.

In addition to considering the affect associated with the low desire, there are two parameters that should be considered in the process of assessing a complaint of low sexual desire. The first is whether the desire problem is present in all situations, or is it specific to one partner or to one environment (e.g., at home but not in a hotel room on vacation)? This is often referred to as *global* versus *specific* dimension. Global desire problems are generally more difficult to treat and usually require a more protracted therapy process.

The second dimension relates to whether the desire problem always existed for an individual, or is it a problem that has followed a period of normal sexual desire? This is referred to as a *primary* (or lifelong) versus *secondary* (also known as learned or acquired) desire problem and, as might be suspected, primary desire problems are much more difficult to treat.

In summary, HSDD occurs in both men and women and is best quantified in terms of sexual interest rather than actual behavior. In addition, this disorder may have a complex etiological picture composed of biological, psychological, social (interpersonal), and cultural ingredients. Finally, the diagnosis depends upon the affective correlates of the low desire report, as well as whether the low desire is specific versus global, and lifelong versus short term.

Mention of how desire disorders may present by men versus women is appropriate to this point. In this regard, it is not uncommon for a man to say, "I have no interest in sex." From such a statement, it is difficult to determine whether he is referring to his low sexual desire, or really talking about his lack of erection. Thus, as clinicians, we need to separate an arousal disorder (see Chapter 3) from a desire disorder. There are several ways this might be done. For example, you might ask the man, "Despite your lack of interest, can you still get an erection?" Obviously, if he can still get an erection, you have ruled out an arousal disorder. Alternatively, you might ask, "Compared to your past, how would you rate your interest in sex?" (If appropriate, you may want to use the word "horniness.") Or you might ask, "Compared to other guys, how horny do you get?" You might also ask, "If you can get an erection, do you think that you would be interested in having sex?" On the basis of the man's answers, you will have to make a judgment regarding whether the disorder involves a desire deficiency or an arousal problem.

When evaluating a woman's low sexual arousal, we usually find it easier to make the distinction between low desire and arousal difficulties, because women tend, on average, to be more in touch with their feelings than are men. Rarely would a woman state, "I have no interest in sex" and mean that she has trouble with her arousal (lubrication). With women, however, this statement may mean that she has aversion to sex; thus, a differential diagnosis between HSDD and SAD is in order according to criteria previously described.

Occasionally, we encounter a situation in which one partner of a couple will present with a complaint of low sexual desire but, after assessment, it is sometimes determined that the more accurate diagnosis is that there is a discrepancy in desire and neither partner has a problem. Most typically, in a heterosexual couple, it is the female partner who presents with low desire in such a scenario. When it is the male partner presenting with low desire, the complaint is most likely secondary to concerns over erectile failure or premature ejaculation rather than to the female partner's greater desire.

The discrepancy may exist because one partner has truly an excessive sexual desire. In some cases, the excess can be of "addictive" proportions yet, interestingly, the person with less desire may be branded as the one with the sexual problem, that is, low desire.

When sexual desire discrepancy problems exist, even when one partner may be characterized as sexually addictive, it is important therapeutically to remove blame, discuss differences, and focus on quality of sexual interactions rather than quantity. When a true addiction or paraphiliac problem exists, treatment should also include a relapse prevention–based approach (Laws, 1989; Laws & O'Donohue, 1997). It is also important to point out to the partner with "excessive desire" that excessive pressure for sex and a constant sense of sexual availability is a sexual turnoff. Such sexual persistence disturbs two important ingredients of sexual desire (i.e., novelty and risk; Stoller, 1975). A recent case from our files illustrates this point.

Mr. and Mrs. Armstrong were each highly successful business executives when they first met 2 years prior to their marriage. When they entered therapy, they had been happily married for 10 years. This was the second marriage for both. Because of their financial success, Mr. Armstrong had encouraged Mrs. Armstrong to retire from her career and oversee the training of their show dogs (a passion for both of them). Mrs. Armstrong agreed to this but felt guilty about her new role, which she saw as being a bit selfish.

The presenting complaint in therapy was that Mrs. Armstrong had lost her sexual desire and wished to "regain" her sex interest. Separate assessment interviews revealed that both partners were respectful and loving to each other but that currently they were having sex only three or four times per week rather than the usual six or seven. Mrs. Armstrong disclosed that she was feeling increasingly upset by her husband's constant sexual advances. She also said that she did not approach him for affection or undress in front of him because such behaviors would immediately lead to sexual pressure. Surprisingly, she identified herself as having a problem with low desire.

Mr. Armstrong revealed in his interview that he was desirous of sex every single day and that whenever he traveled, he hired high-class female escorts for sex. This behavior, which he knew would be hurtful to his wife if she became aware of it, was done secretively. He had, in fact, unsuccessfully tried to control this behavior. In a second solo interview with Mr. Armstrong, he agreed that his sexual desire was excessive and adversely affecting his wife. He further agreed that the focus should be on controlling his sexual acting out with female escorts and reducing the sexual pressure on his wife. Mutual quality rather than quantity became the goal.

Mr. Armstrong chose to disclose his secrets to his wife in the spirit of putting the issues behind them and getting on the right track. Mrs. Armstrong was surprisingly understanding and became a supportive partner for his individual treatment within a relapse prevention model. Six months after treatment, Mr. Armstrong was fully in control of his sexual acting out with escorts and had greatly reduced sexual pressure on Mrs. Armstrong. She was very pleased and felt comfortable approaching her husband for affection and once again enjoyed their sexual encounters.

This case illustrates two points: (1) the value of separate partner assessment interviews, and (2) the inaccuracy of patient self-diagnosis. Although Mrs. Armstrong's level of sexual desire was not dysfunctional or pathological, the decrease in her desire resulted from the cumulative sexual pressure she felt from her husband. The excitement of seducing her husband was lost because he was perpetually interested in sex. This constant sexual availability and demand diminished her desire.

Prevalence

Prevalence data for all categories of sexual dysfunction vary widely across studies (Simons & Carey, 2001); specific prevalence figures are influenced by the population under study and assessment methodology. Nevertheless, it is generally agreed that the prevalence of HSDD has increased over the last few decades (Beck, 1995). One report suggests that the rate in the general population is 5% of men and 22% of women (Laumann, Paik, & Rosen, 1999). The proportion of females to males that present with this problem varies depending on the age of the sample under study. For example, Segraves and Segraves (1991) report that males with a primary diagnosis of HSDD are approximately 11 years older than females presenting with this disorder as a primary diagnosis. Panser et al. (1995) also report a correlation between age and HSDD, such that when patient age was 70 or older, the prevalence rate was 26%.

Studies of the prevalence of HSDD among men in primary care settings yield estimates ranging from a current prevalence of 3% (Jamieson & Steege, 1996) to 55% (Catalan et al., 1992a). In sexuality clinics, prevalence rates tend to be higher (Simons & Carey, 2001). For both men and women, co-occurrence of HSDD with other sexual disorders is common and occurs at a rate of 41% for females and 47% for males (Segraves & Segraves, 1991). Beck (1995) points out that elevated levels of depression, dependence, anxiety, and generalized symptoms of distress are often reported in association with the diagnosis of HSDD in men and women. Three studies examined HSDD in relation to HIV status (Catalan et al., 1992a, 1992b; Pace, Rundell, & Paolucci, 1990). Estimates of current HSDD among HIV-positive persons range from 13% (Pace et al., 1990) to 75% (Catalan et al., 1992b). The most consistently reported comorbid problem, however, seems to be poor dyadic adjustment (Trudel, Boulos, & Matte, 1993). Because poor dyadic adjustment has such a high comorbidity with HSDD, we pay careful attention to the sexual history of the patient to determine whether the low desire problem was a cause of or a result of the dyadic adjustment problem.

Etiology

The etiology of sexual desire disorders in men and women is among the most complex challenges in all sexual dysfunctions. Within all other sexual dysfunction problems, low desire is likely to also be present.

Biological Factors

Biological factors can play an important role in the etiology of low desire disorders for men and women. Any medical condition that causes pain or discomfort may indirectly result in low sexual desire. Age, endocrine imbalance, and some medications may have a more direct impact on sexual desire in men and women. Laumann et al. (1999) found that low desire was much more prevalent in older men (40–70 years). For women, low desire seems to decrease rather than increase with age (Laumann et al., 1999).

The most robust biological factor affecting sexual desire may be hormonal disturbances. For example, men with abnormally low testosterone levels (due to disease) experience low sexual desire and loss of erection (Bancroft, 1988; Benson, 1994). In men whose testosterone level is artificially lowered pharmacologically (as in the treatment of sex offenders), sexual desire also decreases (Bradford, 1997). Men undergoing treatment for prostate cancer who are treated with the testosterone lowering drugs also experience a reducing of sexual desire. Additional evidence of the importance of testosterone on sexual desire in men comes from studies that demonstrate that men with low testosterone, who are treated with exogenous testosterone, increase their sexual desire and erectile capacity (Benson, 1994; Carani et al., 1990).

This same robust phenomenon of hormone levels and sexual desire does not exist as clearly in women. Sherwin (1988) has presented evidence that testosterone level in women is important and can be related to self-reported sexual desire. Beck (1995), however, argues that the evidence of the role of hormones and sexual desire in women is inconsistent. Sarrel (2000) reports that hormone replacement therapy (HRT) can enhance sexual desire in a significant percentage of women but notes that there are other women whose sexual difficulties remain unresponsive to HRT. There also appears to be a significant subgroup of women whose desire difficulties respond initially to HRT but who subsequently revert to their initial problems. Bartlik, Legere, and Andersson (1999) provide evidence that the combined use of sex therapy and HRT can be effective for women with low desire. Much more attention is now being paid to this topic and we are likely to have more information in the next few years regarding the role of hormones in women.

Sexual desire in men and women can also be affected by pharmacological agents used for treating nonsexual disorders. Research has consistently identified the side effect of low desire in response to treatment of depression, phobic disorders, and obsessive–compulsive disorder using selective serotonin reuptake inhibitors (SSRIs; Graziottin, 1998; Kennedy, Dickens, Eisfeld, & Bagby, 1999; Kennedy et al., 2000). Delayed ejaculation is also reported in men on SSRI therapy and clomipramine has been shown in controlled trials to delay ejaculation in men experiencing premature ejaculation and is advised for treating this problem (Segraves, Saran, Segraves, & McGuire, 1993).

The list of pharmacological agents that adversely affect sexual desire in men and women continues to grow. Widely used medications for the treatment of diverse disorders including hypertension, cancer, glaucoma, and seizures have all been reported to reduce sexual desire (Segraves, 1988). It should be remembered that, although the side effects of these medications are frequently reported, there are many individuals taking these medications whose sexual desire is unaffected.

Psychosocial Factors

In cases of secondary HSDD, the low desire is often caused by acute emotional states such as anger, depression, or anxiety (Beck, 1995). Barlow's (1986) theoretical work is important in explaining the effects that emotional states can have on sexual functioning. According to this model, prior history, cognitive set or expectations, and affect combine to yield either a positive or negative sexual response. In addition, there may be some stimuli that have more of a generic or intrinsic ability to affect mood and subsequent sexual response. Barlow's theoretical work and empirical research studies identify mood state as potentially an important etiological factor in low sexual desire in men and women. Certainly, mood that is affected by dyadic conflict or personal tragedy can easily be identified as etiologically contributory to low sexual desire.

Although there are no controlled studies that have looked longitudinally at the psychological etiology of primary low desire, retrospective assessment interviews almost always identify sexual trauma or negative sexual messages as likely childhood sources of this problem. Blatant sexual abuse over time, incidents of sexual assault, warnings or negative messages about sex from parents, lack of affection from parents, or strongly stated religious or moral repression of sex have all been commonly expressed in our cases of primary HSDD. Also, we have often found low self-esteem, especially associated with one's perceived physical undesirability, present in the history of such cases.

Several studies have confirmed the association between history of sexual abuse and desire difficulties. For example, Kinzl, Traweger, and Biebl (1995) assessed 202 female university students (ages 18–30 years) for early familial experience and childhood sexual abuse (CSA), and reported that victims of multiple CSA more frequently reported sexual desire disorders than did single-incident victims and nonvictims. Single-incident victims reported no significantly different rates for any kind of sexual dysfunction. Negative early familial experiences were also related to desire disorders. Results suggest that both family dysfunction and sexual victimization contribute to desire disorders in adulthood.

Sexual functioning and satisfaction will be maximized to the extent that sexual activity occurs in a context of positive expectancies. When individuals fear negative consequences as a result of being sexually expressive, then the risk of a desire disorder increases. This risk is most salient when being sexually active can threaten one's health, one's life, or the life of one's partners, as is the case with HIV. Several studies have documented reduced sexual desire as a function of infecting or becoming infected with HIV or other sexually transmitted diseases (STDs) (e.g., Goggin, Engelson, Rabkin, & Kotler, 1998; Meyer-Bahlburg et al., 1993). Fortunately, there are means to avert infection, and information and skills training can help to restore desire under such circumstances.

A variety of psychiatric conditions are often associated with low desire, including depression, anxiety disorders, posttraumatic stress disorder (Letourneau, Resnick, Kilpatrick, Saunders, & Best, 1996), eating disorders (de Silva & Todd, 1998), and severe mental illnesses such as schizophrenia (Bhui, Puffet, & Strathdee, 1997). Severe psychiatric disorders do not preclude effective sex therapy, but these disorders must usually be addressed first, before the sexual dysfunction.

One other often overlooked contributor to low desire is simply lack of attraction for one's sexual partner. We have encountered numerous cases in which a couple will report complete happiness with each other in all respects, but one partner may not find his or her partner sexually attractive. This may be due to physical changes that a partner has gone through over time (i.e., weight gain) or repeated unrewarding sexual experiences due to a partner's lack of sexual skill or enthusiasm. The net result is low sexual desire.

Desire is likely to be impaired by any number of psychosocial stressors, such as financial difficulties, work stress, or illness. Disappointment associated with infertility can also reduce sexual interest and desire in partners (Herer & Holzapfel, 1993). Laumann et al. (1999) identified a number of important factors of etiological significance in men and women experiencing sexual dysfunction. Emotional stress, deterioration in economic position, lower socioeconomic status, and, more generally, poor quality of life were all identified by these researchers as having important negative associations with sexual well-being.

3

Sexual Arousal Disorders

"Sexual arousal" refers to the physiological, cognitive, and affective changes that serve to prepare men and women for sexual activity. In men, the most conspicuous physiological changes seen during sexual arousal are penile tumescence and elevation of the testes. In our patients' parlance, we are referring to "getting an erection" or having a "hard-on." In women, a more extensive and complex pattern of physiological changes occurs, including vaso-congestion in the pelvis, vaginal lubrication, swelling of the external genitalia, narrowing of the outer one-third of the vaginal barrel, lengthening and widening of the inner two-thirds of the vaginal barrel, and breast tumescence. Clients tend to simplify and summarize these changes as "getting aroused," and their absence as lack of lubrication or vaginal dryness. Although these physiological changes occur both locally and centrally, it is reduced genital arousal that typically brings people to seek professional assistance.

The cognitive and affective components of sexual arousal are more subtle than the physiological one. The cognitive component involves the focusing and narrowing of attention to erotic stimuli (e.g., one's partner), fantasies, and sexual cues (e.g., music, perfume, lingerie). The affective component involves the subjective sense of sexual excitement, novelty, romance, and pleasure that a person experiences concurrently with the aforementioned physiological changes and cognitive focus. In some persons, there can also be an "anxious," edgy, or excited tinge to the affective experience of sexual arousal. In our clinical experience, women tend to be more aware than are men of the cognitive–affective changes associated with sexual arousal.

Although the physiological changes associated with arousal are relatively clear, it can be very challenging to distinguish between diminished subjective arousal (i.e., the cognitive and affective components) and low sexual desire (see Chapter 2). DSM-IV-TR offers no information to aid differential diagnosis in this instance. In our experience, difficulties in sexual arousal can involve the complete absence of these physiological, cognitive, and affective changes. Most commonly, however, arousal disorders can be differentiated from desire disorders by the premature termination or incomplete nature of physiological arousal; that is, individuals may approach the sexual situation eagerly (i.e., they experience sexual desire) but find that they cannot sustain their arousal level to the degree that they would like (e.g., to achieve adequate lubrication or a full erection).

In DSM-IV-TR, arousal difficulties in men are referred to as male erectile disorder; in women, they are called female sexual arousal disorder.

Male Erectile Disorder

Description and Clinical Presentation

In men, inadequate arousal is typically experienced as the partial or complete inability to attain, or to maintain, an erection that is sufficient for intromission and subsequent sexual activity. Erectile disorder may also involve a lessened or absent sense of excitement and pleasure. This difficulty has also been referred to as "erectile dysfunction" (the term that we use), "erectile incompetence," and "impotence." The term "impotence" is no longer preferred because it suggests a global "lack of power" and is thus both imprecise and pejorative. Similarly, "erectile incompetence" is not used because of its obvious negative connotations.

Like other sexual dysfunctions, erectile dysfunction can be further classified as "lifelong" (or "primary") versus "acquired" (or "secondary"), and as "generalized" versus "situational." When erectile dysfunction is characterized as lifelong and/or global, the problem is typically seen as more serious and difficult to treat. The DSM-IV-TR criteria for erectile dysfunction are presented in Table 3.1.

Some men with erectile dysfunction may report that they are completely unable to obtain an erection; however, such complete dysfunction is, in our experience, rare. It is more common for men to report that they are able to obtain a partial erection that is too soft to achieve penetration; alternatively, they may report that they can achieve a full erection but are unable to maintain their erection long enough to permit penetration and intravaginal ejaculation. For some men, the detumescence is extremely rapid and may occur within seconds. Some men report that full erections are possible during noncoital stimulation—for example, during masturbation or nocturnally during rapid eye movement (REM) sleep. The amount of tumescence and rigidity that a

TABLE 3.1. Diagnostic Criteria for Male Erectile Disorder (302.72)

A. Persistent or recurrent inability to attain, or to maintain until completion of the sexual activity, an adequate erection.

B. The disturbance causes marked distress or interpersonal difficulty.

C. The erectile dysfunction is not better accounted for by another Axis I disorder (other than a Sexual Dysfunction) and is not due exclusively to the direct physiological effects of a substance (e.g., a drug of abuse, a medication) or a general medical condition.

Specify type:
  Lifelong Type
  Acquire Type

Specify type:
  Generalized Type
  Situational Type

Specify:
  Due to Psychological Factors
  Due to Combined Factors

Note. From American Psychiatric Association (2000). Copyright 2000 by the American Psychiatric Association. Reprinted by permission.

man achieves may depend upon the extent of physiological involvement (discussed further in the "Etiology" section).

As a result of their erectile difficulties, men often report that they are embarrassed, discouraged, depressed, and even suicidal. Many will have tried several "home remedies" such as self-medication with alcohol or other drugs, viewing erotica, or becoming involved with a different partner. These remedies often fail. Part of the reason why such self-help strategies fail is that men may approach affairs or masturbation under less than ideal conditions; that is, they may often approach masturbation with the same attitude as when with a partner, namely, with a demand to "perform." Thus, the man may masturbate to "see if it works" and may not approach masturbation in a relaxed, erotic way.

Similarly, with a new partner, to "test the waters," a man may be as performance-oriented as with his usual partner and not have the luxury of relaxed, unrestricted time. A failure with a different partner is usually looked upon by such men as additional evidence of their own inadequacy rather than the stress inherent in the situation.

Prevalence

Erectile difficulties seem to be ubiquitous. For some men, they represent a transitory problem, whereas others experience erectile difficulties that are more persistent and troublesome. In either case, it has been estimated that as many as 50% of all men will experience erectile difficulties at some point in their lives (Kaplan, 1974). The commonness of this problem is suggested by several indirect indicators, for example, (1) the number of self-help organizations for men with erectile problems; (2) the numerous advertisements that continue to appear in the so-called "men's magazines" offering magical "cures" of one type or another; and (3) the active and flourishing commercial interest in medical treatments that has, since the launch of Viagra, brought frequent television advertisements to homes throughout the United States.

There has also been a plethora of scientific studies that have investigated the prevalence of erectile dysfunction. We have reviewed this rather large literature for each of the past two decades (Simons & Carey, 2001; Spector & Carey, 1990). Here, we focus our review on the most recent data.

Current (past year) prevalence estimates in the general population range as high as 10% (Laumann et al., 1999) across 10 studies published since 1990. As expected, the prevalence of erectile dysfunction increases with age, history of heart disease, diabetes, treated hypertension, untreated ulcer, arthritis, allergy, and smoking (Feldman, Goldstein, Hatzichristou, Krane, & McKinlay, 1994; Mannino, Klenvens, & Flanders, 1994; Panser et al., 1995; Ventegodt, 1998; Weinhardt & Carey, 1996). Five of these studies have examined current erectile dysfunction in older men in the community (Cogen & Steinman, 1990; Feldman et al., 1994; Jonler et al., 1995; Panser et al., 1995; Schiavi, Mandeli, Schreiner-Engel, & Chambers, 1991). Estimates range from 20% of men reporting erections less than half the time when sexually stimulated in the previous year (Jonler et al., 1995) to 52% of men (Feldman et al., 1994). The estimate by Feldman et al. combines "minimal, moderate, and complete" erectile dysfunction. The prevalence of moderate erectile dysfunction in the sample was 25%.

In primary care settings, current estimates of erectile dysfunction range from less than 1% (Wei et al., 1994) to 37% (Singer, Weiner, & Sanchez-Ramos, 1992) across seven studies. This wide fluctuation can be attributed to differences among assessment criteria and presence of important risk factors in the samples, including advanced age, medications (Read, King, & Watson, 1997), diabetes (Weinhardt & Carey, 1996), and medicated hypertension (Modebe, 1990). The highest rates were reported among patients with Parkinson's disease (60%; Singer et al., 1992) and Alzheimer's disease (55%; Zeiss, Davies, Wood, & Tinklenberg, 1990).

In sexuality clinics, current rates of erectile dysfunction range from 1% (Jindal & Dhall, 1990) to 53% (Bhui, Herriot, Dein, & Watson, 1994) across seven recent studies. The lowest estimate was based upon interviews of women regarding the sexual functioning of both themselves and their male partner. Not one of these studies utilized DSM criteria and few provided operational definitions; thus, it is not surprising that there exists such disparity in prevalence estimates. Goldmeier et al. (1997), Rosser, Metz, Bockting, and Buroker (1997), and Verma, Khaitan, and Singh (1998) may be the most methodologically sound studies and provide current estimates of 19%, 15%, and 24%, respectively. Rosser et al. (1997) report lifetime estimates of 40% (getting an erection) and 46% (maintaining an erection).

Thus, extensive research on the prevalence of erectile dysfunction has yielded a wide range of estimates across samples that vary in age, physical well-being, and other important risk factors. The bottom line from these scientific investigations is that erection problems occur commonly in men in a variety of setting.

Etiology

Because erectile difficulties have been studied more than any other sexual disorder, our understanding of the causes of such problems is more advanced than for other sexual dysfunctions. The current conceptualization of erectile dysfunction has advanced well beyond the "organic" versus "functional" dichotomy that once characterized the field. Well-trained professionals now recognize that the etiology of acquired erectile dysfunction, in most cases, involves a complex interplay of biological, psychological, and social influences (lifelong erectile dysfunction is usually caused by psychological factors). For the interested reader, there are entire books on the subject of erectile dysfunction (e.g., Carson, Kirby, & Goldstein, 1999; Rosen & Leiblum, 1992). It is beyond the scope of this book to review all of the relevant literature, but we have outlined many of the causal agents contributing to erectile dysfunction.

BIOLOGICAL FACTORS

As introduced in Chapter 1, biological factors can be subdivided into indirect and direct factors. Indirect factors are any medical factors that are present but have no direct pathophysiology that causes sexual dysfunction. For example, chronic obstructive pulmonary disease (COPD) does not directly cause sexual dysfunction, but a man with COPD may feel out of breath during sexual activity and his breathlessness may cause worry and result in erectile failure. Direct factors, such as diabetes, cardiovascular disease, and low testosterone, directly inhibit the body's ability to respond sexually. The most important direct medical factors that inhibit male arousal (erections) are endocrinological, cardiovascular, and neurological.

Endocrine deficiencies have long been suspected as a leading cause of erectile difficulties. This notion resulted from early research that established a relationship between low levels of plasma testosterone and erectile capacity (Werner, 1939). More recent work, which is methodologically superior, has provided only mixed support for the hypothesis that reduced testosterone levels are responsible for erectile dysfunction (Jones, 1985). For example, numerous reports document the fact that men with prepubertal levels of serum testosterone can continue to obtain adequate erections (e.g., Davidson, Camargo, Smith, & Kwan, 1983; Heim, 1981). In apparent contrast, other investigators of hypogonadal men have reported increases in the frequency of spontaneous erections following testosterone replacement (e.g., Salmimies, Kockott, Pirke, Vogt, & Schill, 1982). Subsequent, more fine-grained analysis suggests that testosterone may be more important to fantasy-based arousal (and sexual desire) than it is to externally stimulated erections (Bancroft & Wu, 1983).

Further support of this finding comes from research with healthy men with erectile dysfunction. Schiavi, White, Mandeli, and Levine (1977) found that testosterone administration to this population increased sexual activity (sexual desire) but did not enhance erectile capacity.

Low levels of testosterone in men may result in erection problems subsequent to decreases in sexual desire (Rakic, Starcevic, Starcevic, & Marinkovic, 1997). However, testosterone treatment of men with low testosterone does not always reverse the erection problem. In an attempt to predict which men with low testosterone would most benefit from testosterone treatment, Rakic et al. found that higher luteinizing hormone (LH) levels and lower values of the testosterone-to-LH ratio (T/LH) were most significantly associated with good outcome of testosterone treatment. Furthermore, gradual onset of erectile problems and older age were also correlated with positive treatment outcome.

Despite these mixed findings, most experts agree that although hormonal factors can cause erectile dysfunction, they are rarely the sole or primary cause (e.g., Bancroft, 1984; Jones, 1985; Schover & Jensen, 1988).

Vascular diseases and difficulties represent a serious threat to erectile functioning (Papadopoulos, 1989). Because erection is primarily a vascular phenomenon (i.e., erection is achieved by a threefold increase in penile blood flow), malfunctions in either the arterial (i.e., inflow) or venous (i.e., outflow) systems are likely to result in erectile difficulties.

Arterial inflow may be insufficient as a result of any pathological condition that limits the amount of blood reaching the penis; diseases affecting the central pelvic arteries (supplying the legs) and/or the finer arteries (supplying the penis directly) may be implicated. Arteriosclerosis (i.e., thickening, hardening, and loss of elasticity of the wall of the arteries) may be the most common cause of arterial insufficiency (Wagner & Metz, 1981). Ruzbarsky and Michal (1977) completed postmortem investigations of 30 men, ages 19–85, and reported that all men over 38 years of age began to show signs of vascular disease in the penile arteries. The adequacy of the arterial inflow can be assessed with Doppler studies (Jetvich, 1980; see also Chapter 6 for further details), and surgical revascularization interventions are available (see Chapter 8).

In the last decade, surgical revascularization for arterial inflow problems and surgical procedures to correct veno-occlusive dysfunction have improved (Hatzinger, Seemann, Grenacher, & Rassweiler, 1997; Shah & Kulkarni, 1995). Furthermore, long-term studies now point to the benefits of vascular surgery for male erectile dysfunction when cases are carefully and comprehensively screened (Jarow & DeFranzo, 1996; Sarramon, Bertrand, Malavaud, & Rischmann, 1997; Sasso, Gulino, Di-Pinto, & Alcini, 1996).

Neurological disease can also contribute to erectile difficulties. Potential etiological contributors include diseases of the cerebral hemispheres (e.g., epilepsy), the spinal cord (e.g., multiple sclerosis), the peripheral nervous system (e.g., diabetes, renal disease), and trauma (e.g., damage from pelvic cancer surgery or spinal cord injury). The most common neurologically based cause may be diabetes, which places men at high risk for neuropathy and subsequent erectile dysfunction (Weinhardt & Carey, 1996). However, neuropathy is not the only pathogenesis attributed to diabetes. Diabetes not only affects endocrine factors but also vascular factors that in turn can impact on erectile functioning. In a recent review, Ertekin (1998) points out that there are four different types of diabetic erectile dysfunction:

1. Acute–subacute erectile dysfunction indirectly related to diabetes.
2. Chronic–progressive erectile dysfunction directly related to diabetes.
3. Acute–subacute erectile dysfunction directly related to diabetes.
4. Other conditions contributing to or producing erectile dysfunction.

Within each type, the onset and course of erectile dysfunction is different. As is the case with any disease state that might be implicated in sexual dysfunction, prior sexual history and other nonmedical factors must also be considered to obtain an accurate assessment of the sexual problem. For interested readers, Ertekin (1998) provides a concise and comprehensive review of the role of diabetes in sexual dysfunction for men and women.

Alcohol has long been known to impair male sexual arousal (penile rigidity and orgasm) as blood alcohol levels increase (Cooper, 1994). However, as Langevin et al. (1985) have pointed out, the pure physiological affects of acute alcohol ingestion on erectile functioning are difficult to determine because alcohol often enhances desire that may compensate for any degradation of physiological capability. In an attempt to tease out the pure physiological impact of acute alcohol ingestion on erectile capacity, Cooper (1994) looked at the impact of alcohol on nocturnal penile tumescence (NPT). Using RigiScan measures on a single subject, Cooper concluded that alcohol ingestion suppresses REM and thus delays NPT responding, but only at high dosages does alcohol impair erectile capacity. Individual differences will, of course, determine the impact of acute alcohol ingestion on sexual functioning, but in general, low levels of alcohol do not appear to impair erectile capacity physiologically. In fact, alcohol at low levels is reported to have enhancing effects on sexual arousal/desire, but this may be due to expectancy as much as any specific pharmacological mechanism (Roehrich & Kinder, 1991). Acute alcohol ingestion in association with sexual behavior is undoubtedly widespread. Laumann, Gagnon, Michael, and Michaels (1994) have found that about 9% of men and 6% of women report "frequent" ingestion of alcohol before or during sex.

Chronic alcohol abuse is much more likely to impair sexual functioning due to actual damage to the body. Neuropathy as well as testicular and liver damage occur as a result of chronic alcoholism. For men, liver and testicular damage result in lowered testosterone levels and possible gynecomastia (breast growth).

Fahrner (1987) reported the results of a study of 116 patients in an alcohol treatment program in Germany. Twenty-three patients (20%) reported frequent episodes of erectile dysfunction, and 26 patients (22%) reported very frequent or continuous episodes of erectile dysfunction. Fahrner also cited numerous other studies documenting the higher prevalence of erectile dysfunction among chronic alcoholics.

The effects of other substances of abuse on erectile functioning are less well studied (Buffum, 1986). It has been suggested that the frequency of erectile dysfunction among heroin users is 28–43% and among methadone users, is 40–50% (Segraves, Madsen, Carter, & Davis, 1985); both estimates are considerably higher than the frequency found in the general population. Reliable estimates are not available for other commonly abused substances (e.g., amphetamines, marijuana, cocaine). The illicit status of these drugs makes well-controlled studies in humans very challenging. Thus, we recommend strongly that your assessment include careful attention to substance use for all patients.

Numerous prescribed medications are implicated as causes of sexual dysfunction in both men and women (Crenshaw & Goldberg, 1996). Most consistently reported, however, are the antidepressant medications. In a review, Margolese and Assalian (1996) reported the effects of various antidepressants on the sexual functioning of men and women. They concluded that for sexual arousal, the tricyclic and tetracyclic antidepressants are most likely to impair erections and vaginal lubrication. SSRIs may also impair arousal but are most often associated with delays in orgasm.

Antihypertensive medications have also been implicated in impairment of erectile functioning (Bansal, 1988; Moss & Procci, 1982; Papadopoulos, 1989; Segraves et al., 1985). Critical examination of the research on this topic, however, finds few studies that provide support for this belief. In one of the methodologically strongest studies, Rosen, Kostis, and Jekelis (1988) investigated, prospectively, the effects of four beta-blockers (Atenolol, metoprolol, pindolol, and propranolol) on sexual functioning in 30 healthy men. Over a

70-day period, the subjects received each of the four drugs and a placebo, and assessment of erectile functioning was obtained with measures of NPT. The results indicated that only minor, clinically insignificant decrements in tumescence were observed.

Additional studies on other antihypertensive agents have similarly revealed clinically insignificant impact on erectile functioning (Broekman, Haensel, Van de Ven, & Slob, 1992; Morrissette, Skinner, Hoffman, Levine, & Davidson, 1993). The evidence for suppression of erectile functioning associated with antihypertensive agents is not impressive (Rosen, Kostis, Jekelis, & Taska, 1994).

PSYCHOSOCIAL FACTORS

Numerous psychological factors have been linked with erection problems. Negative affect, particularly anxiety, has been suggested as an etiological factor by several theorists. For example, Kaplan (1974) has stated that performance anxiety "almost invariably contributes to impotence" (p. 129). Similarly, Masters and Johnson (1970) highlighted the "profound role played by fears of performance" (p. 84). Meisler and Carey (1991) found that acute depressed affect (not to be confused with the clinical syndrome of major depression) could also reduce subjective arousal.

The work of Barlow and his colleagues (e.g., Barlow, Sakheim, & Beck, 1983; Beck, Barlow, & Sakheim, 1983; Sakheim, Barlow, Beck, & Abrahamson, 1984) has been especially instrumental in delineating important psychological factors related to erectile failure. In an ingenious series of studies, they have compared men experiencing erectile failure to men not experiencing any erectile problems and have found that men who experience erectile disorder tend to:

- underestimate the amount of erection they are actually achieving, whereas functional men are more accurate in their estimation of arousal;
- increase their erection response when they focus on nonerotic stimuli, whereas men who experience no erectile failure tend to decrease their erection response when they focus on nonerotic stimuli following arousal;
- decrease their erection response when demands to get aroused are made, whereas functional men experience the opposite; and
- display negative affect in the presence of erotic stimulation.

In a review of the empirical research, Barlow (1986) concluded that cognitive interference and negative affect specific to sexual stimuli are central to erectile dysfunction.

Weisberg, Brown, Wincze, and Barlow (2000) have added a new dimension to our understanding of the impact of psychological factors on male erectile response. In a study of healthy males, Weisberg et al. exposed men to erotic tapes while recording subjective arousal and physiological measures of penile circumference change. Men were then given false feedback stating that their sexual response was less than what was typical. Half of the subjects were told that the reason for their poor performance was most likely due to the poor quality of the videos (external attribution), and half were told that their poor performance was predictable because of personality characteristics regarding sexuality (identifying with questionnaires completed by the subjects, i.e., internal attribution). Subjects given the internal attribution showed less penile response than subjects given the external attribution, even though both groups were equal in previous video exposures. These results suggest that a self-critical attributional style may be one important factor contributing to erectile response in men. Ongoing research will determine if women also show similar decrements in arousal depending on attributional style.

Psychosocial stress may also play an important role in the erectile difficulties of some men. In one study, the effects of chronic (i.e., actual or threatened unemployment) and acute (i.e., giving a speech about their sexual behaviors) stress were evaluated (Morokoff, Baum, McKinnon, & Gillilland, 1987). The results suggested that erectile impairment occurs as a result of a combination of chronic and acute stress.

Relationship factors have been implicated by so many writers (e.g., Kaplan, 1974) that their importance may seem obvious. Certainly, one would expect that a man must be comfortable with his partner if he is to become aroused. McCabe and Cobain (1998) reported that dysfunctional men are more likely than sexually functioning males to report deficits in both the sexual and nonsexual aspects of their current relationship, and the dysfunctional males reported more frequent arguments.

In a very creative and interesting study, Speckens et al. (1995) explored relationship and sexual attitudes, sexual functioning, and psychological adjustment of female partners of two groups of men with erectile dysfunction (ED): those for whom no organic cause could be found and those with organically-based ED. Female partners of men without purported psychogenic ED reported higher levels of sexual interest, more relationship problems, and a higher instance of vaginismus and dyspareunia than did female partners of men with organic ED. Female sexual dysfunctions in the group without organic ED usually preceded onset of erectile difficulties. This study is one of the few that examines the relationship dynamics, or comorbidity, of male and female sexual dysfunction.

Clinical experience suggests that anger toward one's partner, or being in a relationship that is not characterized by trust, is a risk factor for ED. Relationships characterized by critical interactions are also believed to place men at greater risk for erectile difficulties.

Female Sexual Arousal Disorder

Historically, less attention has been paid to female sexuality issues than to male sexuality issues but, with the much publicized success of Viagra for men, increased attention has been focused on female arousal concerns. This attention has been reflected in both multidisciplinary scientific meetings (O'Leary & Rosen, 1998) and the popular press (Leland, 2000). Although the number of research studies devoted to female sexuality still lags far behind research for men, there are signs of increased scientific study. Several important research contributions have occurred over the past 10 years (Laan, 1994; Meston & Gorzaka, 1996; Meston, Gorzaka, & Wright, 1997; Palace, 1995a, 1995b; Palace & Gorzalka, 1990).

Description and Clinical Presentation

Female sexual arousal disorder refers to a lack of responsiveness to sexual stimulation in women. Previously, disorders of female sexual functioning (including desire, arousal, and orgasmic disorders) were grouped into the global category of "frigidity." The term "frigidity" is imprecise in that it does not distinguish among the three stages of sexual functioning, and it is pejorative; consequently, it is no longer used by most sex therapists.

Physiologically, female sexual arousal disorder is characterized by the absence of vaginal lubrication and expansion. In contrast to erectile dysfunction, these signs may go undetected or unreported by a woman, and by her partner. Subjectively, this disorder is accompanied by a failure to find pleasure in sexual activities and by a lack of erotic feelings. (Here, the distinction between female sexual arousal disorder and hypoactive sexual desire disorder [see Chapter 2] can become blurred.) Like other sexual dysfunctions, female sexual arousal disorder can be classified as "lifelong" or "acquired," and as "generalized" or "situational." The DSM-IV-TR criteria for female sexual arousal disorder are presented in Table 3.2.

Tollison and Adams (1979) suggest that a woman is not as likely as a man to show an extremely negative response to an arousal disorder. These authors suggest that women may respond with an array of feelings, ranging from casual acceptance to mild anxiety or depression. Compared to the more extreme reaction of men to ED, this lessened emotional response may reflect a kind of sexual "learned helplessness" (see Seligman, 1975); that is, women have traditionally been discouraged from seeking pleasure from sex, and thus are less likely to complain when their pleasure is compromised. Alternatively,

TABLE 3.2. Diagnostic Criteria for Female Sexual Arousal Disorder (302.72)

A. Persistent or recurrent inability to attain, or to maintain until completion of the sexual activity, an adequate lubrication–swelling response of sexual excitement.

B. The disturbance causes marked distress or interpersonal difficulty.

C. The sexual dysfunction is not better accounted for by another Axis I disorder (except another Sexual Dysfunction) and is not due exclusively to the direct physiological effects of a substance (e.g., a drug or abuse, a medication) or a general medical condition.

Specify type:
  Lifelong Type
  Acquired Type

Specify type:
  Generalized Type
  Situational Type

Specify:
  Due to Psychological Factors
  Due to Combined Factors

Note. From American Psychiatric Association (2000). Copyright 2000 by the American Psychiatric Association. Reprinted by permission.

because women can bypass their arousal problem (i.e., by using a vaginal lubricant) much more easily than men, it may be that women's arousal problems have received less attention (Schover & Jensen, 1988). Furthermore, a man's response is essentially a public event, that is, both he and his partner are aware of the problem, whereas a woman's arousal problem may be unknown to her partner and to her (especially if a lubricant is used).

Prevalence

Studies that delineate the prevalence of sexual dysfunction in women are still rare. During the past 10 years, however, there have been several important population-based studies that greatly add to our knowledge base.

Rosen, Taylor, Leiblum, and Bachmann (1993) examined the sexual functioning of 329 healthy women, ages 18–73, enrolled in a Women's Wellness Center. Using vaginal lubrication as the best indicator of sexual arousal, 43% of all women reported at least occasional lubrication problems. Lack of lubrication during intercourse increased with aging, since 52% of women above age 50 reported at least occasional vaginal dryness compared to 38% of women under 50. Lack of lubrication on 50% or more occasions was reported by 14% of all women. A second, larger study of sexual dysfunction in the United States was conducted by Laumann et al. (1999) on a sample of 1,749 women between the ages of 18 and 59. In this sample, 14% of women were identified with sexual arousal disorder.

In studies conducted outside the United States, Lindal and Stefansson (1993) reported a lifetime prevalence of 6% in a large random sample of 55- to 57-year-old women in Iceland, whereas Fugl-Meyer and Sjogren Fugl-Meyer (1999) reported a 1-year prevalence of 8% in a Swedish sample that ranged in age from 18 years to 74 years. Lack of standard criteria across studies and sampling differences make the large disparities across studies difficult to interpret.

Chandraiah, Levenson, and Collins (1991) reported a lifetime prevalence of female sexual arousal disorder among 21% of their sample from a primary care setting based upon DSM-III criteria. In a small study that examined women attending a sex therapy clinic in India (Verma et al., 1998), no cases of female dysfunctions were reported. Clearly, more research on the prevalence of arousal disorders in women is needed.

Etiology

Compared to male arousal disorder, considerably less research has been conducted on the etiology of female sexual arousal disorder.

BIOLOGICAL FACTORS

Impairments to either the vascular or neurological systems are likely to cause arousal difficulties. For example, pelvic vascular disease can result in lowered vaginal lubrication (Schover & Jensen, 1988); similarly, neurological impairment secondary to diabetes (Spector, Leiblum, Carey, & Rosen, 1993) or multiple sclerosis may also impair arousal (e.g., Hulter, 1999; Schreiner-Engel, Schiavi, Vietorisz, Eichel, & Smith, 1985). Hormonal changes, especially decreases in estrogen, can also increase vaginal dryness and may lead to dyspareunia (see Chapter 5). Such changes are likely following menopause or oophorectomy, or during lactation. Unfortunately, there is only limited information on the sexuality of older women (Gentili & Mulligan, 1998).

As with males, there is evidence that prescription drugs, especially the SSRIs, impair sexual functioning in women (Bartlik, Kaplan, & Kaplan, 1995; Segraves, 1995). There is also evidence that oral contraceptives may adversely impact female sexual arousal. As with any medication, there is great individual variability, and some women may experience prosexual consequences of SSRIs and oral contraceptives.

There is also evidence that some drugs enhance sexual arousal, providing indirect evidence of the importance of biological factors. For example, Meston and Heiman (1998) investigated the effects of ephedrine sulfate, an alpha- and beta-adrenergic agonist, on subjective and physiological sexual arousal in 20 women. They found that ephedrine significantly increased vaginal pulse amplitude responses to erotic films; despite this effect, there was no effect on subjective ratings of sexual arousal. They concluded that ephedrine can facilitate the initial stages of physiological sexual arousal in women.

PSYCHOSOCIAL FACTORS

A large number of psychological factors have been hypothesized as possible impediments to female arousal. Anger, depression, low self-esteem, performance anxiety, worry, and sexual abuse are some examples of these factors. Laan (1994) has pointed out that women may downplay their subjective reports of sexual arousal. Furthermore, she suggests, women may not be accurate perceivers of their sexual arousal, and thus may not attend carefully to initial genital sensations of arousal. Tollison and Adams (1979) also identified a number of psychological states (doubt, guilt, fear, shame, conflict, embarrassment, tension, disgust, irritation, resentment, grief) as possible causes of arousal difficulties in women.

The research on psychological factors has focused on emotional, cognitive, and experiential factors. Morokoff and Heiman (1980) compared 11 women seeking treatment for female sexual arousal disorder to 11 normal control subjects. Both groups viewed an erotic film, listened to an erotic audiotape, and engaged in sexual fantasy while physiological and subjective arousal were monitored. Contrary to expectation, the two groups did not differ in their physiological response to erotic stimuli; however, dysfunctional subjects did rate their subjective arousal as less than that of the control group. The authors concluded that cognitive and emotional factors are important in understanding female sexual arousal disorder.

Beggs, Calhoun, and Wolchik (1987) isolated the effects of a particular affective state (anxiety) on arousal. To do this, they compared sexual arousal occurring during sexual anxiety stimuli to that occurring during sexual pleasure stimuli in 19 sexually functional women. Although both sets of stimuli enhanced arousal, increases in the pleasure condition were greater than those during the anxiety condition. Dunn, Croft, and Hackett (1999) provided data based on survey responses from 979 women (ages 18–75 years) in England. They found that anxiety and depression were both associated with arousal problems in women.

The importance of cognitive and affective factors was confirmed in a study by McCabe and Cobain (1998), who evaluated the relative contribution of attitudinal and emotional factors to sexual dysfunction in a large sample of sexually functional and dysfunctional adults (ages 25–68 years). Results indicated that dysfunctional women were more likely than their functional counterparts to report negative attitudes toward sex during adolescence and currently, and to acknowledge performance anxiety concerns.

Clinical experience suggests that history of sexual abuse may be an important etiological factor (Becker, 1989). McCabe and Cobain (1998) found that dysfunctional women were more likely than their functional counterparts to report sexual abuse during adolescence. Sarwer and Durlak (1996) investigated 359 married adult women (ages 20–65 years) who sought sex therapy with their spouses. Women whose abuse history involved sexual penetration were signficantly more likely to experience sexual dysfuntion. A number of other studies have repeatedly indicated that a history of childhood sexual abuse (CSA) is not unusual for women who report a sexual dysfunction (Hirst, Baggaley, & Watson, 1996; Kinzl et al., 1995; Mullen, Martin, Anderson, Romans, & Herbison, 1994). In our experience, the arousal dysfunction may be specific to the type of abuse that occurred. For example, a woman who was abused by her step-father by fondling may be responsive to kissing and intercourse but nonresponsive to petting and foreplay. In other instances, the arousal dysfunction may be more global. Thus, careful and sensitive assessment of prior sexual experiences is warranted.

While recognizing the traumatic effects of CSA, it is important to point out that not all women who were sexually abused as children (or adults) will develop sexual difficulties. For example, Greenwald, Leitenberg, Cado, and Tarran (1990) studied 54 women (ages 23–61 years) who had been sexually abused as children. These women were matched with 54 nonabused controls. Although abused women reported more psychological symptoms, they did not differ from controls on self-reported levels of sexual satisfaction or sexual dysfunction. Other studies (e.g., Kinzl et al., 1995) have documented that characteristics of the abuse experience (e.g., involving penetration or not, involving a family member, multiple vs. single episodes) may moderate the impact of the sexual abuse experience.

Several relationship factors have been hypothesized as causes of female sexual arousal disorder, including lack of adequate stimulation by male partners and poor communication. Although the importance of such factors may seem obvious, little research has been completed. In one study reported by McCabe and Cobain (1998), dysfunctional women were more likely than functional controls to report deficits in both the sexual and nonsexual aspects of their current relationship. Dunn et al. (1999) found that marital difficulties were the best predictor of sexual arousal difficulties in a stratified random sample of 979 women in England.

We also completed a study that explored sexual satisfaction among women as a function of partner understanding and communication (Purnine & Carey, 1997). Partners from 76 cohabitating heterosexual couples independently completed measures of their own and their partners' sexual preferences, sexual and general relationship adjustment, sexual difficulties, marital role preferences, depression, and social desirability. Results indicated that women's sexual satisfaction was associated with both men's understanding of women's preferences and preference agreement.

4

Orgasmic Disorders

Men's and women's orgasmic experiences, like roller coasters, range on a continuum from mild to extreme ("unbelievably pleasurable," "exhausting, out of control release"). Depictions in popular literature and movies tend to emphasize the high points, whereas reports from our patients tend to evidence the low ones. Although we do not consider orgasm to be the *raison d'etre*, the be-all-and-end-all of sexual functioning, many people do.

Often, patients will present with concerns about the absence of coital, multiple, or simultaneous orgasms; they feel disappointed that they cannot achieve what "everyone else" enjoys, and they seek a cure of their "deficits." Male patients have presented to us their concerns about "premature ejaculation" when, in fact, they are exceeding all textbook definitions. One recent male patient stated that he has never had a problem bringing any female partner to orgasm through intercourse, that he usually lasted 5–10 or more minutes with vigorous thrusting and often has multiple intercourse experiences during sexual episodes. Still, he felt he had a "premature ejaculation" problem because he would ejaculate before he wanted to on some occasions and "guys in the porno movies could hold it to the exact moment they wanted, no matter how intense the sex was." As discussed in the treatment chapters, such patients often benefit from some gently delivered education supplemented with normative data and reassurance regarding their sexual health.

Because men's orgasms are almost always coincident with observable ejaculate, most men have little doubt about the occurrence of their orgasm (even if it is very mild). Women, on the other hand, without the observable feedback of ejaculation, are at times unsure as to whether or not they have had

39

an orgasm. In this regard, it is important to know that many women do not regularly experience coital orgasms (Kaplan, 1989); that is, such women do not reach orgasm *solely* through intercourse, because the stimulation obtained by penile thrusting is not intense and direct enough to produce an orgasm. This is not a "dysfunction"—it is natural and normal. To repeat: The absence of orgasm during intercourse is not a sexual dysfunction! Even the women who do experience orgasm during intercourse may not have an orgasm during every "coital connection" (to use Master and Johnson's terminology).

Similarly, simultaneous orgasms make for excellent drama on the silver screen (or on the home-based DVD) but such sexual synchrony occurs only rarely for most couples. Finally, multiple orgasms do occur, but they are relatively infrequent and occur only for a minority of women and men. For example, Kinsey, Pomeroy, Martin, and Gebhard (1953) reported that 14% of their female sample were capable of multiple orgasms on some occasions. More recent evidence presented by Dunn and Trost (1989) suggests that some men do not always experience detumescence following an orgasm, and that they have been able to experience a series of orgasms.

For many people, however, orgasm never occurs, it occurs only after prolonged stimulation, or it occurs with such rapidity that it causes concern for both partners. Thus, in this chapter we discuss the one female and the two male complaints about the orgasmic phase: female orgasmic disorder, male orgasmic disorder, and premature ejaculation.

Female Orgasmic Disorder

Description and Clinical Presentation

Female orgasmic disorder is the DSM-IV-TR term that was formerly listed as inhibited female orgasm. This recognized, common disorder occurs mainly in younger women. In DSM-IV-TR, female orgasmic disorder is a persistent or recurrent delay in, or absence of, orgasm following a normal sexual excitement phase (Criterion A). Criterion B is that the disorder causes stress or interpersonal difficulty, and Criterion C is that the disorder is not better accounted for by another Axis I disorder, substance use or abuse, or a general medical condition such as diabetes (see Table 4.1).

DSM-IV-TR has not eliminated the possibility of gender bias in the therapist's judgment of the adequacy of sexual stimulation.

On the one hand, some women who do not achieve orgasm may experience sexual desire, feelings of increasing sexual arousal and sexual satisfaction. On the other hand, other women who do not achieve orgasm may judge their sexual experience with bitterness and disappointment. The interpretation of anorgasmia as acceptable or unacceptable may be influenced by numerous

TABLE 4.1. Diagnostic Criteria for Female Orgasmic Disorder (302.73)

A. Persistent or recurrent delay in, or absence of, orgasm following a normal sexual excitement phase. Women exhibit wide variability in the type or intensity of stimulation that triggers orgasm. The diagnosis of Female Orgasmic Disorder should be based on the clinician's judgment that the woman's orgasmic capacity is less than would be reasonable for her age, sexual experience, and the adequacy of sexual stimulation she receives.

B. The disturbance causes marked distress or interpersonal difficulty.

C. The orgasmic dysfunction is not better accounted for by another Axis I disorder (except another Sexual Dysfunction) and is not due exclusively to the direct physiological effects of a substance (e.g., a drug of abuse, a medication) or a general medical condition.

Specify type:
  Lifelong Type
  Acquired Type

Specify Type:
  Generalized Type
  Situational Type

Specify:
  Due to Psychological Factors
  Due to Combined Factors

Note. From American Psychiatric Association (2000). Copyright 2000 by the American Psychiatric Association. Reprinted by permission.

psychological factors (i.e., knowledge, self-esteem, self-confidence) as well as interpersonal factors (i.e., partner pressure, knowledge, or satisfaction).

Crooks and Baur (1996) point out that most therapists do not consider it a problem if women enjoy intercourse but only experience orgasm through direct clitoral stimulation. In fact, the absence of orgasm during intercourse without direct clitoral stimulation is common. It is unhelpful and heterosexist to suggest that the only valid orgasm is one achieved through penile–vaginal intercourse.

Prevalence

It is interesting to review the scientific literature for this dysfunction over time. In the earliest published study conducted with the general population, Kinsey et al. (1953) found that 10% of all women reported that they had never experienced orgasm. Twenty years later, Levine and Yost (1976) reported that 5% of their subjects were anorgasmic, perhaps indicating a decrease over time in the number of women who had never experienced orgasm. Other studies conducted in the 1970s, which focused on women who never or infrequently experienced orgasm, the rates ranged from 15% to 20% (Ard, 1977; Athanasiou, Shaver, & Tavris, 1970; Hunt, 1974).

More recent studies, conducted during the 1990s, continue to provide a wide range of estimates, depending upon sampling strategy, definitional criteria, and assessment interval. For example, studies from three northern European countries obtained prevalence rates that ranged from 4% to 7% (Ernst, Foeldenyi, & Angst, 1993; Lindal & Steffansson, 1993; Ventegodt, 1998). In the United States, a recent report indicates that 24% of women have been unable to reach orgasm for several months over the past year (Laumann et al., 1999), whereas a population-based, random sample of 349 women (ages 51–61 years) in Massachussetts yielded a rate of 10%. Overall, population studies over the years in a variety of countries have yielded estimates ranging from 4% to 24%; if we assume this range contains the true estimate, we are left to conclude that many women experience difficulty in achieving orgasm. Indeed, this conclusion is supported by epidemiological evidence from clinical settings.

Results from recent studies in primary care populations estimate the prevalence of female orgasmic disorder between 5% (Chandraiah et al., 1991) and 42% (Read et al., 1997). Rosen et al. (1993) studied women in an outpatient gynecological clinic in the United States, and reported that 15% of these patients experienced difficulty in achieving orgasm. Prevalence estimates obtained in sexuality clinics tend to be even higher, with estimates of 22% (Goldmeier et al., 1997) and 41% (Jindal & Dhall, 1990). Thus, women who experience orgasmic difficulties have often sought professional assistance.

A final note regarding prevalence is that the available research suggests that unmarried women are more likely to experience dysfunction (Kinsey et al., 1953), as are women of lower socioeconomic status (SES; Levine & Yost, 1976). Hite (1976) reported that whereas only 4% of women are anorgasmic during masturbation, as many as 70% are anorgasmic during coitus.

Etiology

BIOLOGICAL FACTORS

Morokoff (1978) provided an early overview of the determinants of female orgasm. Among the biological variables she identified, the condition of the pubococcygeal musculature seemed to be the one most likely to be associated with female orgasmic disorder. Subsequent research, however, has challenged her conclusion. Chambless et al. (1982) investigated the relationship of pubococcygeal condition to orgasmic responsiveness in 102 nonclinical subjects. Contrary to expectation, pubococcygeal strength was not associated with frequency or self-reported intensity of orgasm. Moreover, women with greater pubococcygeal strength did not report that vaginal stimulation contributed more to the attainment of orgasm; nor did these subjects rate vaginal sensations during intercourse as more pleasurable. A follow-up intervention study (Chambless et al., 1984) supported these earlier findings. In the 1984 study, females with a low frequency of coital orgasm were taught to use Kegel exercises to improve their pubococcygeal strength, and despite a significant increase in strength, no improvement in coital orgasmic frequency was observed.

A more recent review by Heiman (2000) identified a number of neurophysiological factors that have been implicated as potential causes of orgasmic difficulties; she notes that any disease, injury, or disruption that affects the sympathetic or parasympathetic nervous systems might impair orgasm in women. Goldstein and Berman (1998) suggest that atherosclerotic vascular disease may be a common cause.

The effects of hormonal variation on orgasm are also unclear, especially in older women. Sherwin (1985) studied 8 women who had been maintained on a combined estrogen–androgen drug since undergoing hysterectomy (i.e., removal of the uterus) and bilateral oophorectomy (i.e., removal of the ovaries) 2 years previously. Although hormone replacement did influence sexual desire and arousal, rates of orgasm were unchanged. Similar findings were reported by Sherwin, Gelfand, and Brender (1985). However, in a third study, Sherwin and Gelfand (1987) found that orgasmic rates were enhanced following the administration of the estrogen–androgen preparation.

Ample evidence now documents negative effects of pharmacological medications on orgasmic functioning in women. Treatment with the SSRIs commonly result in anorgasmia in women at follow-up evaluations (Crenshaw & Goldberg, 1996; Labbate, Grimes, & Arana, 1998; Margolese & Assalian, 1996; Shen & Hsu, 1995), although the mechanisms are not well understood (Meston & Gorzalka, 1992).

Fortunately, it appears that the side effects of some SSRIs and other psychoactive medications can be countered medically. For example, in one study, a 35-year-old woman with recurrent depressive illness was treated with sertraline and responded to the drug but complained of persistent loss of orgasmic quality and frequency (Grimes & Labbate, 1996). Her orgasms did not improve during a 2-week trial of cyproheptadine but, when treated with an injection of adjunctive bupropion, she reported a spontaneous orgasm. Another case study documented that treatment of an anxiety disorder with paroxetine led to anorgasmia of over 1 year's duration (Ashton, 1999); in this case, the woman's anorgasmia improved following treatment when sildenafil citrate (Viagra) was taken 1 hour prior to anticipated sexual activity. The benefits of this medication have been replicated in several other recent studies (Nurnberg, Hensley, Lauriello, Parker, & Keith, 1999; Salerian et al., 2000).

There is evidence that the use of alcohol and other drugs may interfere with orgasmic functioning. Wilsnack (1984) reviewed the literature to determine the relationship between alcohol consumption and sexual dysfunction. On the basis of numerous clinical reports and laboratory research, she concluded that rates of orgasmic disorder are higher in alcoholic women compared to rates found among normative samples (i.e., Kinsey et al., 1953). Among the better studies she reviewed was one conducted by Malatesta, Pollack, Crotty, and Peacock (1982), who investigated the effect of acute intoxication on female orgasmic response. The results indicated that higher blood alcohol concentrations were associated with longer orgasmic latencies and decreased subjective intensity of orgasm.

The potential influence of chronic illness on orgasmic functioning, especially in older women, has also been investigated. With a large sample of young female diabetics (mean age 33 years) and controls, Kolodny (1971) found that 35% of female diabetics had orgasmic dysfunction compared to 6% of controls; in all cases, the orgasmic dysfunction occurred after the diagnosis of diabetes. More recently, Hulter (1999) has provided an excellent series of studies researching the impact of diabetes, multiple sclerosis, and various hypothalamo-pituitary disorders (HPD) on female sexual functioning. She has found higher rates of anorgasmia in women with diabetes (14%), multiple sclerosis (51%), and HPD (69%) compared to the relatively low rate of 2% in healthy female controls.

PSYCHOSOCIAL FACTORS

The search for psychological factors associated with female orgasmic disorder has often focused, unfortunately, on personality characteristics rather than cognitive and affective factors. For example, in two early studies, women with orgasmic dysfunction were found to have a psychological profile characterized by high levels of distress (Derogatis & Meyer, 1979; Derogatis, Meyer, & King, 1981); however, great heterogeneity in symptom distress was evident. Therefore, in a later study (Derogatis, Fagan, Schmidt, Wise, & Gilden, 1986), two subtypes of orgasmic dysfunction were identified. One subtype included women who were relatively well informed about sexuality, possessed more liberal sexual attitudes, had higher levels of desire, and reported a richer fantasy life. Derogatis et al. (1986) speculated that the etiology of orgasmic dysfunction in these women was more likely to involve either biological or interpersonal factors. In contrast, the second subtype included women who possessed feelings of inferiority, negative body images, and higher levels of psychological symptoms. The authors speculated that the principal etiology for this subtype was psychogenic.

Interesting research has begun to examine the effect of distraction on orgasm in women. In one study, Dove and Wiederman (2000) surveyed 74 young women regarding cognitive distraction and their sexuality. Those women who reported greater cognitive distraction during sexual activity with a partner also reported relatively lower sexual esteem, less sexual satisfaction, less consistent orgasms, and higher incidence of pretending orgasm.

Former relationships may continue to exert a negative influence on orgasm in women. There is some evidence that having a history of sexual abuse may lead to orgasmic difficulties in some women (Norris & Feldman-Summers, 1981; Tsai, Feldman-Summers, & Edgar, 1979). Fisher (1973), in his classic study and book, *The Female Orgasm*, found that early abandonment by an important male figure was consistently found among anorgasmic women.

Clinicians have long recognized the important role of a woman's current relationship as well, and some research has confirmed these beliefs. For example, McGovern, Stewart, and LoPiccolo (1975) compared 6 cases of lifelong orgasmic disorder with 6 cases of acquired orgasmic disorder. These two groups did not differ with regard to age, overall physical health, length of married life, or most aspects of sexual behavior. Two important differences did emerge. First, women with the acquired disorder were much more dissatisfied with their marital relationships than were women with the lifelong disorder. Second, women with acquired orgasmic disorder had an established and constrained pattern of orgasmic "release"; that is, most of these women could reach orgasm through one narrowly constrained method of masturbation. The authors suggested that this pattern may have been maladaptive, especially with regard to treatment-assisted change.

Kilmann et al. (1984) compared 48 couples in which the woman had acquired orgasmic disorder to 63 sexually satisfied couples. Compared to satisfied couples, couples with orgasmic disorder reported greater dissatisfaction with the frequency and range of their sexual activities. Within the dysfunctional group, males reported low self-acceptance as well as low mate acceptance; females reported lower self-acceptance. Males in the dysfunctional couples also exhibited less accurate knowledge of their partners' sexual preferences.

Two more recent studies have also explored current relationship patterns. Hawton, Gath, and Day (1994) found that frequency of orgasm was associated with better marital adjustment. In a fine-grained analysis, Purnine and Carey (1997) reported that communication patterns, and especially men's understanding of their partner's sexual preferences, were an important predictor of sexual satisfaction. Little research has directly evaluated the obvious hypotheses of sexual skills in partners, or sexual attraction to partners, nor has anyone, to our knowledge, explored Apfelbaum's (2000) notion that some people can have a "autosexual orientation" that might constrain orgasms during dyadic behavior.

Larger social influences are undoubtedly relevant to women's sexual functioning, including orgasmic experiences. It is not surprising, but interesting nonetheless that in her early review, Morokoff (1978) found that the most significant influence on women's orgasmic functioning was decade of birth! That is, she found that being born later in the 20th century was related to higher frequency of orgasm! This certainly suggests that changing social norms, associated with the general movement toward greater equality for women, may be an important social factor. More recently, Laumann et al. (1994) provided evidence that SES and educational level were related to a woman's orgasmic experience. Women with lower SES and less education were less likely to experience orgasm.

Male Orgasmic Disorder

Description and Clinical Presentation

What do the terms "blue balls," "dry runs," "aspermatism," "ejaculatory incompetence," "retarded ejaculation," "absence of ejaculation," "ejaculatory impotence," "ejaculatory inhibition," and "inhibited male orgasm" have in common? All of these phrases have been used to describe the problem some men have in reaching orgasm. Rather than refer to such patients' difficulty as "retarded," "incompetent," "impotent," or "inhibited," all of which have either a pejorative or a theoretical slant, we prefer to use the new DSM-IV-TR label "male orgasmic disorder," or simply to describe the problem directly and without inference as "delayed or absent male orgasm."

Male orgasmic disorder refers to the persistent difficulty or inability to achieve orgasm despite the (apparent) presence of adequate desire, arousal, and stimulation (see Table 4.2). Most commonly, however, the term refers to a condition in which a man is not able to ejaculate with his partner, even though he is able to achieve and maintain an erection. Importantly, the man is typically able to ejaculate during masturbation or sleep (nocturnal emissions or "wet dreams.") Like other sexual dysfunctions, male orgasmic disorders can be lifelong or acquired, and generalized or specific.

It is important to distinguish between male orgasmic disorder and "retrograde ejaculation." The latter difficulty occurs as a result of some medications (e.g., anticholinergic drugs), after some (but not all) prostate surgeries, and occasionally as a consequence of diabetic neuropathy. With retrograde ejaculation, a man does ejaculate and experience orgasm, but the ejaculatory fluid travels backward (into the bladder) rather than forward and out the urethra. The sensation of orgasm is preserved for most men who experience retrograde ejaculation, although some do report a slight diminution in pleasurable sensation.

It is also important to distinguish between emission and ejaculation. Ejaculation has three stages: (1) emission, (2) bladder neck closure, and

TABLE 4.2. Diagnostic Criteria for Male Orgasmic Disorder (302.74)

A. Persistent or recurrent delay in, or absence of, orgasm following a normal sexual excitement phase during sexual activity that the clinician, taking into account the person's age, judges to be adequate in focus, intensity, and duration.

B. The disturbance causes marked distress or interpersonal difficulty.

C. The orgasmic dysfunction is not better accounted for by another Axis I disorder (except another Sexual Dysfunction) and is not due exclusively to the direct physiological effects of a substance (e.g., a drug of abuse, a medication) or a general medical condition.

Specify type:
Lifelong Type
Acquired Type

Specify Type:
Generalized Type
Situational Type

Specify:
Due to Psychological Factors
Due to Combined Factors

Note. From American Psychiatric Association (2000). Copyright 2000 by the American Psychiatric Association. Reprinted by permission.

(3) ejaculation proper (Segraves et al., 1985). Emission refers to the release of the ejaculate into the pelvic urethra; this release is caused by the contraction of the vas deferens, seminal vesicles, and smooth muscle of the prostate. Bladder neck closure prevents retrograde ejaculation. Finally, ejaculation proper results from contractions of the bulbocavernosus, ischiocavernosus, and urethral muscles (Segraves et al., 1985).

Although no data are available, our clinical impression is that men who experience orgasmic disorders express greater upset than women who experience anorgasmia. The reason for this may be because men expect orgasm to occur 100% of the time they engage in sexual behavior, whereas women's expectations allow for a wider variety of outcomes. Thus, for men, the lack of orgasm, in spite of adequate erotic stimulation, is more likely to be distressing.

Prevalence

Male orgasmic disorder is relatively rare. Studies from the late 1970s provided population estimates that ranged from 4% to 10% (Frank et al., 1978; Nettelbladt & Uddenberg, 1979). More recent population estimates completed in the 1990s have tended to be lower, ranging from 0% (Schiavi et al., 1995) to 3% across six studies (Fugl-Meyer & Sjogren Fugl-Meyer, 1999; Lindal &

Stefansson, 1993; Singer et al., 1992; Solstad & Hertoft, 1993; Ventegodt, 1998). An exception to these rates is the 8% rate reported by Laumann et al. (1999). Estimates from eight primary care samples across four studies range from 0% (Catalan et al., 1992a) to 36% (El-Rufaie et al., 1997), with a median of 9% (Shahar et al., 1991).

In sex therapy settings, male orgasmic disorder may be the dysfunction least often encountered. Masters and Johnson (1970) reported only 17 cases of male orgasmic disorder out of 448 male sexual dysfunction cases they assessed and treated in an 11-year period. Kaplan (1974) stated that her sample size was too insignificant to report. Apfelbaum (2000) notes that he has seen 34 men in his practice but does not provide the total number of patients. Other clinical studies suggest that the dysfunction accounts for 3–8% of the cases presenting for treatment (Bancroft & Coles, 1976; Frank, Anderson, & Kupfer, 1976; Hawton, 1982; Renshaw, 1988). A higher estimate was reported by Frank et al. (1976), who found that 17% of males seeking marital therapy were diagnosed as experiencing male orgasmic disorder.

Estimates from four more recent studies in sexuality clinics report current prevalence estimates from 0% (Bhui et al., 1994) to 38% (Catalan et al., 1992b). One study reported a lifetime prevalence of 39% in gay men (Rosser et al., 1997). Estimates from samples of gay men were notably higher than other samples (i.e., Catalan et al., 1992b; Rosser et al., 1997). Two studies report an increased prevalence (20–38%) of male orgasmic disorder among men with HIV (Catalan et al., 1992a, 1992b).

As this literature review suggests, estimates have ranged widely. It is clear that there have been many methodological differences across these studies, especially involving sampling (e.g., HIV-infected vs. healthy samples) and, most importantly, the definition of the disorder (Simons & Carey, 2001). There has been little agreement regarding whether the delayed or absent orgasm was a single occurrence. Rarely have investigators reported whether the men studied can experience orgasm through masturbation.

Etiology

There has been no systematic research on the cause(s) of male orgasmic disorder. Instead, the literature contains numerous case studies, each of which puts forth its own etiological formulation. Nonetheless, we identify some of these hypotheses and summarize current research.

BIOLOGICAL FACTORS

Munjack and Kanno (1979) reviewed the medical literature for possible drug-related etiologies and identified over 20 different drugs that have been associated with this disorder. Primary culprits include the anticholinergic, anti-adrenergic, antihypertensive, and psychoactive drugs.

PSYCHOSOCIAL FACTORS

At the psychological level of analysis, the possible etiologies that have been identified include fear (of castration, pregnancy, or commitment), performance anxiety and "spectatoring," strict religious proscriptions leading to guilt or avoidance, previous sexual traumas, and hostility (toward one's partner or oneself). Thus, it appears that there may be many pathways to male orgasmic disorder. Indeed, after reviewing the psychosocial literature, Shull and Sprenkle (1980) concluded: "If the literature is searched long enough, almost any and every psychological problem can be associated with [male orgasmic disorder]" (p. 230). Despite the richness of these clinical hypotheses, virtually no systematic research has been conducted on the individual or relationship factors described earlier.

Relationship factors have also been implicated in male orgasmic disorder. A man may be ambivalent about his commitment to the relationship, or he may be anorgasmic as a way of assuming power in a troubled relationship. Shull and Sprenkle (1980) suggest that a simpler relationship problem may also be common, namely, inadequate stimulation. They suggest that the partners may not have created the proper ambience, are using inadequate stimulation techniques, or are engaged in sexual behavior that has lost its erotic impact.

Perhaps the most intriguing explanation for male orgasmic disorder comes from Apfelbaum (2000), who argues that this disorder is more appropriately considered a desire disorder or even a different sexual orientation. He presents anecdotal evidence to support the view that even though men with this disorder can achieve an erection ("automatic erections," in his terms), they are not truly "aroused" or even desirous of partnered sex. Instead, the men have an autosexual orientation (similar to a heterosexual or homosexual orientation), in which they prefer manual stimulation by their own hand rather than partnered sex (of any kind). Contrary to the view that such men are selfish, he argues that they are overly concerned with pleasing their partners and, as a result, tend to focus on their partner's pleasure during coital sex and are distracted from their own sensations.

Premature Ejaculation

Description and Clinical Presentation

Some men complain that they arrive at orgasm too rapidly. What is "too rapidly"? In some cases, ejaculation occurs before the man has entered his partner. Obviously, in heterosexual couples, this would be a serious problem if conception were the goal. In other cases, the man ejaculates "shortly after" penetration. Because the latter phrasing is still imprecise, several theorists have attempted to develop a more precise definition. For example, Master and Johnson (1970) suggested that premature ejaculation be diagnosed when a man "cannot control his ejaculatory process for a sufficient length of time during intravaginal containment to satisfy his partner in at least 50 percent of their coital connections" (p. 92). The problem with this definition is that a large percentage of women cannot reach orgasm through intercourse regardless of how long it lasts! It also inaccurately assumes that this problem occurs only in heterosexuals.

It is very clear that a universally accepted definition of premature ejaculation has not been agreed upon. In a review of the literature, Metz, Pryor, Nesvacil, Abuzzahab, and Koznar (1997) point out that the time to ejaculation after penetration is not a useful criterion for defining premature ejaculation, because this time varies from 1 minute to 10 minutes in published studies. DSM-IV-TR has avoided using objective criteria and has relied on clinical judgment to make the determination (Table 4.3).

In addition to the differences of opinion regarding definition, another debate involves whether premature ejaculation should even be considered a dys-

---

TABLE 4.3. Diagnostic Criteria for Premature Ejaculation (302.75)

A. Persistent or recurrent ejaculation with minimal sexual stimulation before, on, or shortly after penetration and before the person wishes it. The clinician must take into account factors that affect duration of the excitement phase, such as age, novelty of the sexual partner or situation, and recent frequency of sexual activity.

B. The disturbance causes marked distress or interpersonal difficulty.

C. The premature ejaculation is not due exclusively to the direct effects of a substance (e.g., withdrawal from opioids).

Specify type:
Lifelong Type
Acquired Type

Specify Type:
Generalized Type
Situational Type

Specify:
Due to Psychological Factors
Due to Combined Factors

Note. From American Psychiatric Association (2000). Copyright 2000 by the American Psychiatric Association. Reprinted by permission.

function. As noted by Kinsey, Pomeroy, and Martin (1948), the majority of mammals ejaculate at intromission or shortly thereafter. Interviews conducted by Kinsey's group indicated that 75% of their sample of over 6,000 men ejaculated within 2 minutes of vaginal containment. On the basis of these two sources of information, Kinsey and his colleagues went on to suggest that from an evolutionary perspective, such a quick and intense ejaculatory response was probably adaptive and, in this sense, "superior." More recently, a similar position has been argued by Hong (1984), who, after reviewing the literature, concluded that "premature ejaculation by itself should not be of clinical concern unless it is extreme, such as occurring before intromission" (p. 120). To those who might ask about the partner's pleasure, Hong went on to say that "sexual fulfillment in women can be achieved by other and perhaps better means." Although this definition is heterosexist, the key point is that PE may be seen as "adaptive" in a certain sense; thus, we need to be cautious about calling it a dysfunction.

These debates, notwithstanding, many men are troubled by premature ejaculation, and this difficulty can have a destructive effect on a man, his partner, and their relationship (see Case 7 in Chapter 9). Kaplan (1989) suggests that premature ejaculators are at risk for developing a general sense of inadequacy and failure, depression, and other sexual dysfunctions (e.g., desire and erection difficulties). Some men may not understand why they experience premature ejaculation and make inappropriate inferences about their difficulty, such as "I must really be selfish."

Although most women enjoy foreplay and direct clitoral stimulation, others believe that coital stimulation is "better," or that intercourse is the only acceptable form of sexual activity. Such women might be disappointed by, and may lose interest in, sexual intercourse. Partners, too, can make inappropriate inferences (e.g., "I must not be very attractive if he wants to get it over so quick" or "He does not love me"). It is not difficult to see how such outcomes, especially if combined with other expectations and concerns, can have undesirable effects on a relationship. Male partners (men who have sex with other men) experiencing premature ejaculation have expressed similar inferences.

Yet another side effect of premature ejaculation is that a man may try to prolong his "staying power" by any of several home remedies. Some may try to postpone orgasm by holding back, physically or emotionally. Others will try to distract themselves from their pleasurable sensations by thinking of financial concerns or other difficulties. A few may apply anesthetic creams, multiple condoms, or mechanical devices to their penises in an effort to deaden their physiological sensitivity. These "solutions" may have iatrogenic effects and may also lead to erectile problems.

Overall, premature ejaculation can have far-reaching and negative consequences.

Prevalence

As with all of the other sexual dysfunctions we have discussed, the prevalence of premature ejaculation is difficult to determine. Nevertheless, it is typically cited as being the most common sexual dysfunction (e.g., Kaplan, 1974). Recent estimates of PE in the general population provide current (last year) estimates that range from 4% (Ernst et al., 1993; Fugl-Meyer & Sjogren Fugl-Meyer, 1999) to 5% (Schiavi, 1995; Ventegodt, 1998) across three studies. Two additional studies report significantly higher 1-year estimates of 14% (Solstad et al., 1993) and 29% (Laumann et al., 1999). The reason for these discrepant estimates is not clear. Schiavi et al. (1995) report a current estimate of 20% among former alcohol-dependent men.

In primary care settings, current estimates range from 2% (Nirenberg et al., 1991) to 31% (Read et al., 1997) across four studies. The lowest estimate was among alcohol-dependent individuals choosing not to participate in additional research that would have involved intrusive measurements. Volunteers for the study reported a prevalence of 24% (Nirenberg et al., 1991). Thus, prevalence of premature ejaculation may be estimated at between 4% (Catalan et al., 1992b) and 31% (Read et al., 1997).

There is an extremely large range of estimates of the current prevalence of premature ejaculation in sexual health clinic samples. Malatesta and Adams (1984) indicate that 60% of the men entering sex therapy did so with the presenting problem of premature ejaculation. More recently, Metz et al. (1997) concluded that PE is the most common male sexual dysfunction and empirical estimates range from 0% (Bhui et al., 1994; Catalan et al., 1992b) to 77% (Verma et al., 1998) across five studies. The highest estimate (77%; Verma et al., 1998) is from a northern Indian population. This figure is nearly four times the next highest estimate of 22% (Goldmeier et al., 1997). If the estimate of Verma et al. (1998) is considered an outlier, a more accurate range is 0% (Bhui et al., 1994; Catalan et al., 1992b) to 22% (Goldmeier et al., 1997). Laumann et al. (1994) found a prevalence rate of 29%.

Two asides occur to us at this point. The first is based on an empirical finding; that is, Frank et al. (1978) found that 11% of the women in their sample reported that they reached orgasm "too quickly." However, we have no "premature female orgasm" in DSM-IV-TR or other diagnostic schemes. Perhaps this is because women can continue coitus after orgasm; indeed, because they have no equivalent of "refractory period" that most men experience, they may even experience additional orgasms. In contrast, men are less likely to be able to continue intercourse once they have ejaculated, because detumescence is likely. The second aside involves one unanticipated benefit of aging; that is, there is a tendency for young men to ejaculate quickly, and the prevalence of premature ejaculation is believed to decrease with advancing age (Masters & Johnson, 1970).

Etiology

Several hypotheses have been proffered to explain how premature ejaculation may develop.

BIOLOGICAL FACTORS

As already mentioned, premature ejaculation may reflect a physiological characteristic that was formerly adaptive and has been preserved through evolution. This characteristic might be expressed as a kind of "hypersensitivity" to penile stimulation (e.g., Assalian, 1988; Damrav, 1963). In a controlled study, Rowland, Cooper, Slob, Koos, and Houtsmuller (1997) compared physiological and subjective measures of arousal and ejaculation between heterosexual men experiencing premature ejaculation and control male subjects with no ejaculation problems. Premature ejaculators were diagnosed on the basis of their self-reported distress over their inability to control ejaculation during coitus. Specifically, all of these men reported ejaculation latencies of 1 minute or less and fewer "thrusts to ejaculation" than men without premature ejaculation. Using vibrotactile stimulation (a minivibrator attached to the penis) and erotic videotapes, subjective and physiological measures were recorded. The results demonstrated that men with premature ejaculation reported feeling less control over ejaculation when stimulated; indeed, more men in the premature ejaculation group ejaculated (than did men in the control group) under these laboratory conditions. These results suggest possible physiological and cognitive differences in the two groups.

Metz et al. (1997) also provide support for the hypothesis that premature ejaculation results from both biological and psychological factors. Furthermore, within each of these etiological domains, there are multidetermined processes. Metz et al. summarize the neuropharmacological evidence for a biological etiology of premature ejaculation as follows:

1. Ejaculation appears to be inhibited by centrally acting dopamine receptor blockers known as neuroleptics or antipsychotics.
2. Ejaculation appears to be inhibited by increasing the level of serotonin by blocking the reuptake of serotonin. Anecdotal reports also indicate, however, that several SSRIs may, on very rare occasions, precipitate spontaneous orgasm.
3. Ejaculation appears to be inhibited by tricyclic agents that have anticholinergic and alpha-adrenergic antagonistic properties and increase the level of serotonin and norepinephrine by blocking their reuptake. The effect on ejaculation appears dose-related.
4. Ejaculation appears to be minimally inhibited by gamma-aminobutyric acid (GABA)-enhancing agents such as the anxiolytic benzodiazepines, and the effect may be dose related.

5. Ejaculation also appears to be delayed by alpha-adrenergic blockers thought to interfere with sympathetic nervous system activation of the ejaculatory reflexes, such as phenoxybenzamine. Alpha blockage may be the mechanism responsible for this finding.

These effects appear to be single aspects of what must be a multidetermined process of ejaculation, thought to be mediated by both sympathetic and para-sympathetic innervation. The implications from these studies are that (1) both the central and the peripheral nervous system influence ejaculation, and (2) several neurological mechanisms are active in ejaculation. Given these, it is likely that several mechanisms of physiologically induced premature ejaculation may exist (Metz et al., 1997).

PSYCHOSOCIAL FACTORS

Misunderstandings or ignorance about sexual physiology, poor sexual skills, masturbation history, unrealistic expectations, anxiety, and depression have all been posited as possible causes of premature ejaculation. Alternatively, premature ejaculation may reflect a man's poorly developed sensory awareness; that is, regardless of his genital sensitivity, the man with premature ejaculation may fail to develop an appreciation of when he is close to the point of ejaculatory inevitability (Kaplan, 1989). Another view is that premature ejaculation develops as a result of numerous adolescent/young adult practices (e.g., visiting a prostitute who encourages ejaculatory rapidity, having sex in the backseat of a car or other settings not conducive to relaxed lovemaking) that condition a rapid ejaculatory response (Masters & Johnson, 1970).

Some clinicians have suggested that premature ejaculation may result from a lack of sexual or communication skills, interpersonal conflicts or misunderstandings, deficits in managing sexual stimulation, and overall dyadic problems. Little research is available to support or refute these hypotheses.

5

Sexual Pain Disorders

A short story written by Wiseneberg (1996) tells the story of Ruthie, a 35-year-old mother of two who is married to Ruben. Ruthie has experienced pain with sexual intercourse, which she believes occurs because she is overweight. Ruthie describes herself as a something of a contradiction because she has too narrow a vaginal opening to permit intercourse despite her large body. She was able to give birth but has difficulty with penetration during intercourse. Ruthie's story is not unique. In this chapter, we consider two related disorders: dyspareunia and vaginismus. Both can involve actual or feared genital pain and present unique diagnostic challenges.

Dyspareunia

Description and Clinical Presentation

"Dyspareunia" is derived from the Greek word, *dyspareunos*, which means "unhappily mated as bedfellows." This euphemism is currently used, however, to refer specifically to a recurrent pattern of genital pain that occurs before, during, or after coitus. The criteria for DSM-IV-TR diagnosis of dyspareunia are presented in Table 5.1.

Most commonly, the pain is experienced during intercourse, as was the case for Ruthie. Like other dysfunctions, dyspareunia may be characterized as lifelong or acquired, and as generalized or situational. Dyspareunia is more common in women than in men (Masters & Johnson, 1970).

The traditional conceptualization of dyspareunia has been challenged in recent years. Binik and his colleagues point to continuing controversy and

TABLE 5.1. Diagnostic Criteria for Dyspareunia (302.76)

A. Recurrent or persistent genital pain associated with sexual intercourse in either a
   male or a female.

B. The disturbance causes marked distress or interpersonal difficulty.

C. The disturbance is not caused exclusively by Vaginismus or lack of lubrication,
   is not better accounted for by another Axis I disorder (except another Sexual
   Dysfunction), and is not due exclusively to the direct physiological effects of a
   substance (e.g., a drug of abuse, a medication) or a general medical condition.

Specify type:
  Lifelong Type
  Acquired Type

Specify type:
  Generalized Type
  Situational Type

Specify:
  Due to Psychological Factors
  Due to Combined Factors

Note. From American Psychiatric Association (2000). Copyright 2000 by the American Psychiatric Association. Reprinted by permission.

lack of clarity in describing this disorder (Bergeron et al., 1997; Binik,
Bergeron, & Khalifé, 2000; Meana & Binik, 1994; Meana, Binik, Khalifé, &
Cohen, 1997b). Part of the problem, they argue, is that most researchers simply ask patients if they have pain during or after intercourse. Such broad-based
questioning does not yield descriptions of the variations of this disorder that
women experience. The reported presence of pain during penetration attempts
or partial penetration can obfuscate a clear differential diagnosis between
dyspareunia and vaginismus. What is needed is a more detailed assessment of
the pain, including its location, quality, correlates, time course, intensity, and
meaning (Binik et al., 2000).

Dyspareunia in males is seen less commonly by sex therapists. Painful
intercourse in males can occur as a result of some medical conditions. For example, Peyronie's disease is a condition in which plaques develop on the
midshaft of the penis, typically in middle-aged and elderly men, causing
penile narrowing at the point of the plaque and bowing in the penis. Manipula-
tion of the penis through intercourse or masturbation may result in penile pain.
Although this condition may spontaneously remit in some cases, for many
who experience Peyronie's disease, there is no reliable cure.

Other medical conditions that may cause penile pain, such as prostatitis
or urinary tract infections but, in these conditions, the pain occurs most commonly in connection with urination rather than sexual activity. Men may expe-

rience testicular pain in connection with ejaculation. In these cases (which are rare) the pain may be due to an obstructed ejaculatory duct. It is rare for a man to experience testicular pain just in connection with sex and not at other times. Complaints of testicular pain, not exclusively connected to sexual activity, may be due to a variety of factors. Because of the sparse literature on dyspareunia in men, most of our discussion in this chapter focuses on dyspareunia in women.

Pain is a subjective experience that eludes careful measurement and description. Thus, many different accounts of the phenomenology of dyspareunia are available. Abarbanel (1978) suggests that these accounts may be summarized into four categories: (1) perception of a momentary, sharp pain of varying intensity; (2) intermittent painful twinges; (3) repeated intense discomfort; and/or (4) an aching sensation. The pain may also be described as superficial or deep. In addition to the immediate discomfort and the accompanying distress this causes, dyspareunia places a woman at risk for the development of vaginismus (discussed later), as well as secondary desire, arousal, and orgasmic dysfunctions.

Complaints of sexual pain during intercourse present a challenging diagnosis for health care professionals. Clearly, differential diagnosis must begin with a thorough physical examination by a competent physician. A large number of physical factors (see "Etiology") must be assessed and ruled out prior to embarking upon a psychosocially oriented intervention. However, as Masters and Johnson (1970) point out,

> Even after an adequate pelvic examination, the therapist frequently cannot be sure whether the patient is complaining of definitive but undiagnosed pelvic pathology or whether, as has been true countless thousands of times, a sexually dysfunctional woman is using the symptomatology of pain as a means of escaping completely or at least reducing markedly the number of unwelcome sexual encounters in her marriage. (pp. 266–267)

In some cases, it will be possible to identify a clear precipitant, but in most, it will have to be assumed that a combined etiology is operative.

Prevalence

The prevalence of dyspareunia is difficult to determine. In recent studies, prevalence estimates range from 3% (Lindal & Stefansson, 1993; Ventegodt, 1998) to 18% (Moody & Mayberry, 1993) in the general population. This relatively large range is difficult to explain in terms of methodological differences, with the only consistent difference being that the lower estimates tend to be from northern European countries, whereas the higher ones are from the United States (Simons & Carey, 2001).

In an informative study, Glatt, Zinner, and McCormack (1990) surveyed 313 women, most of whom were reported to be in their early 30s. Thirty-nine percent of their sample reported that they had never had dyspareunia. More surprising, however, were the findings that 28% of the women had had dyspareunia at some point in their lives but that it had resolved, and that 34% still had dyspareunia. Of these, nearly half reported that they had had dyspareunia for their entire active sex lives! Many of the women with dyspareunia had not discussed this problem with a professional, and most were unaware of the cause of their difficulty.

In primary care settings, current estimates range from 3% (Heisterberg, 1993) to 46% (Jamieson & Steege, 1996) across the studies reviewed by Simons and Carey (2001). Jamieson and Steege (1996) report point prevalence in a large primary care sample of "pain during or after intercourse." The high prevalence in this and the Weber, Walters, Schover, and Mitchinson (1995) sample (41%) are three times greater than the next highest estimate of 14% (Heisterberg, 1993). These high estimates may be due to the operational definition of the disorder. The DSM-IV-TR diagnostic criteria exclude pain that is associated exclusively with lack of lubrication or vaginismus. Neither of these high estimates exclude pain secondary to these causes. In fact, Weber and colleagues (1995) specifically include vaginal dryness as a sufficient criterion. The range of estimates obtained illustrate the differences that result from nonstandard definitions and the importance of clearly specifying the definitions used.

Nusbaum, Gamble, Skinner, and Heiman (2000) reported the results of a mail survey that they conducted with 964 of 1,480 women who sought routine gynecological care from departments of family practice, and obstetrics and gynecology. The outcomes of interest were self-reported sexual concerns and women's experiences with discussing these concerns with a physician. In this large sample, 75% reported concerns about inadequate lubrication and 72% reported concerns with dyspareunia.

Reports from sexual health care settings have provided prevalence estimates in women ranging from 3% (Hawton, 1982) to 5% (Renshaw, 1988). In a study conducted in Tehran (Iran), Shokrollahi, Mirmohamadi, Mehrabi, and Babaei (1999) reported that 10% of a sample of 300 healthy young, married women reported dyspareunia. Jindal and Dhall (1990) report a current prevalence of 13% in an infertility clinic in India. Compared to the community estimates cited earlier, this lower clinical rate suggests that women may be somewhat disinclined to seek treatment for sexually related pain; alternately, women may be more likely to interpret pain as a "medical" symptom, and to report it to a physician rather than to a sex therapist. Indeed, this latter hypothesis was supported by Burnap and Golden (1967), who found that dyspareunia was commonly reported to general practitioners, and by Steege (1984), who suggests that painful intercourse is the most common sexual complaint received by obstetricians/gynecologists.

Older women have been a population in which dyspareunia has been a focus of research. There is evidence that dyspareunia is more prevalent in postmenopausal women (Rekers, Drogendijk, Valkenburg, & Riphagen, 1992). Prevalence estimates in community samples of postmenopausal women range from 2% (Barlow et al., 1997) to 21% (Wasti, Robinson, Akhtar, Khan, & Badaruddin, 1993).

Consistent with the trends seen in the research literature, anecdotal reports from clinicians also suggest an increase in the prevalence of dyspareunia (Meana & Binik, 1994). Our own experience would support this trend, which may be due to emerging expectations that sex should be enjoyable and that discomforts can be treated or minimized.

Compared to the report of pain associated with sex in women, pain disorders among men appear to be less prevalent (Fass, Fullerton, Naliboff, Hirsch, & Mayer, 1998). Bancroft (1989) and Diokno, Brown, and Herzog (1990) reported prevalence estimates of 1% of the men seen in their clinics. Estimates across seven studies range from a lifetime prevalence of 0.2% in a random population sample (Lindal & Stefansson, 1993) to a lifetime prevalence of 8% in a combined community and clinical sample (Metz & Seifert, 1990). The AIDS pandemic has increased research on the sexual functioning of gay and bisexual men. In one study that examined painful insertive and receptive anal sex in gay men (Rosser et al., 1997), current prevalence estimates of 3% (insertive) and 16% (receptive) were reported.

Etiology

BIOLOGICAL FACTORS

As suggested earlier, many biological factors must be considered when assessing dyspareunia. Abarbanel (1978) divided such factors into three categories: anatomical, pathological, and iatrogenic. Anatomical factors are congenital factors such as genital malformations that contribute to painful intercourse; pathological factors are acute and chronic disease states such as urinary tract infections; and iatrogenic factors are conditions that may result from other medical procedures such as episiotomy.

Bancroft (1989) suggests that an important and often overlooked cause of dyspareunia is tender scarring following either episiotomy or vaginal repair operations. Among the many other candidates are hymenal remnants, the presence of a pelvic tumor, prolapsed ovaries, endometriosis, and pelvic inflammatory diseases.

Binik et al. (2000) argue that there may be several types of dyspareunia, caused by different factors. One type they recognize results from vulvar vestibulitis, a condition that involves multiple tiny erythematous sores in the vulvar vestibule (Bergeron et al., 1997; Nunns & Mandal, 1997; White & Jantos, 1998). Women with this condition report intense superficial pain. The etiology of vulvar vestibulitis itself remains a subject of research interest; however, surgery combined with sex therapy has been successful in selected cases (Bergeron et al., 1997).

A second type of dyspareunia might result from vulvar or vaginal atrophy, perhaps resulting from decreasing estrogen levels postmenopausally. Indeed, in postmenopausal women, women using oral contraceptives, and pregnant women, hormonal changes (i.e., decreased estrogen) may lead to reduced vaginal lubrication and resultant soreness and irritation during penetration (Reamy & White, 1985; Wallis, 1987). We also know cancer treatments that involve radiation to the pelvis and/or removal of the ovaries also reduce estrogen production and increase the risk of dyspareunia. Obviously, mental health professionals are not qualified to evaluate such conditions, but such assessments should constitute part of a comprehensive biopsychosocial intake.

A recent study used vaginal plethysmography to determine whether the psychophysiology of women with dyspareunia ($n = 18$) differs from that of women without dyspareunia ($n = 16$) during sexual arousal (Wouda et al., 1998). Women in both groups demonstrated an increase in vaginal vasocongestion while watching erotic scenes compared to a rest condition. Interestingly, when the participants watched videos depicting cunnilingus and fellatio, the reactions were equivalent across the two groups. However, when participants watched videos showing vaginal intercourse, there was a further increase in vaginal vasocongestion in the women without dyspareunia but a decrease in vasocongestion in women with dyspareunia.

PSYCHOSOCIAL FACTORS

A useful categorization of psychological influences on dyspareunia has been presented by Lazarus (1988), who divided these factors into three categories: developmental, traumatic, and relational. Developmental factors are learned attitudes, such as painful expectations conveyed by a parent; traumatic factors are sex experience that caused upset, such as rape; and relational factors are experiences that may be specific to one or more partners, such as very unskilled approaches to sex.

Psychosocial problems may lead to a complaint of coital pain or exacerbate preexisting discomfort. Individual risk factors such as anxiety, fear, and depression, as well as religious orthodoxy, decreased self-esteem, and poor body image, have all been suggested (Reamy & White, 1985). Interpersonal factors, including anger at one's partner, inadequate communication, and distrust, should also be considered. Moreover, dyspareunia may be most likely to occur in couples in which the male partner is unassertive and accommodating. Thus, such couples' transactional style may place them at risk. (We do not mean to imply that women with dyspareunia should be treated more forcefully by their partners; we do wish to suggest that the overly sensitive nature of the partners in these cases may be worth noticing.)

Whenever there is a complaint of genital pain, especially in the absence of confirmed organic pathology, you need to determine whether your patient might be a survivor of sexual abuse or trauma. Complaints of pain during intercourse or other sexual activity can be an important sign of such a history (Golding, 1996; Keane, Young, & Boyle, 1996). Meana, Binik, Khalifé, and Cohen (1999) studied 100 women (mean age 38 years) with dyspareunia and found that the women who made psychosocial attributions regarding their condition reported higher levels of psychological distress, lower levels of marital adjustment, and more frequent reports of sexual assault.

We want to end this brief review of the literature by citing additional work reported by Meana and colleagues (1997a, 1997b). In one study, these authors found that dyspareunic pain was experienced by women in a number of anatomical locations, that penetration was not required, and that psychosocial variables had no predictive value. They discussed how women who experience dyspareunia often go back and forth between physicians and mental health care providers, do not receive benefit, and often feel sexually inadequate. They argued for a paradigm shift in dyspareunia research from its current conceptualization as a sexual dysfunction to a conceptualization as a pain problem. This view, although nontraditional, is one that deserves increased attention.

Vaginismus

Description and Clinical Presentation

"Vaginismus" is usually defined as the involuntary spasm of the pelvic muscles located in the outer third of the vaginal barrel; the muscle groups affected include the perineal muscles and the levator ani muscles, although in severe cases the adductors of the thighs, the rectus abdominis, and the gluteus muscles may also be involved (Lamont, 1978; American Psychiatric Association, 1994). DSM-IV-TR criteria for vaginismus stipulate further that the spasms be recurrent or persistent and interfere with intercourse (see Table 5.2).

The DSM-IV-TR classification of vaginismus does not mention pain as a criterion for classification, but vaginismus is often discussed in the literature as a severe case of dyspareunia (Meana & Binik, 1994). In spite of this defini-

TABLE 5.2. Diagnostic Criteria for Vaginismus (306.51)

A. Recurrent or persistent involuntary spasm of the musculature of the outer third of the vagina that interferes with sexual intercourse.

B. The disturbance causes marked distress or interpersonal difficulty.

C. The disturbance is not better accounted for by another Axis I disorder (e.g., Somatization Disorder) and is not due exclusively to the direct physiological effects of a general medical condition.

Specify type:
  Lifelong Type
  Acquired Type

Specify type:
  Generalized Type
  Situational Type

Specify:
  Due to Psychological Factors
  Due to Combined Factors

Note. From American Psychiatric Association (2000). Copyright 2000 by the American Psychiatric Association. Reprinted by permission.

tion and the lack of pain as a descriptive criterion, vaginismus is included in this chapter because, clinically, women most often either fear or actually experience pain upon penetration. Furthermore, the treatment strategy for both vaginismus and dyspareunia in women is often similar (see Chapter 7).

Typically, the muscle spasms occur in anticipation of intercourse or during intromission. Thus, when penile penetration is attempted, women and their partners report that the sensation is as if "the penis hits a 'brick wall' about one inch inside the vagina" (Lamont, 1978, p. 633). However, spasms may also occur during pelvic or self-examination; in extreme cases, this reflex contraction may follow attempts to insert anything into the vagina, including tampons, fingers, or a speculum.

Distinguishing vaginismus from dyspareunia, sexual aversion disorder, and even hypoactive sexual desire disorder can be difficult. Thus, we do *not* recommend that diagnosis be made solely on the basis of patient or partner report. Instead, we encourage confirmation of this dysfunction by pelvic examination, performed by a physician (preferably an experienced and sensitive female gynecologist). The primary purpose of this examination is to rule out organic pathology. However, it can also be useful to demonstrate the global nature of the response. It is extremely important that a patient find a gynecologist who will discuss the purpose of the gynecological examination and not further traumatize the patient but be willing to approach her in a desensitization model over several visits if necessary. At any rate, although the examination should be approached with as little pressure as possible, it is necessary at some point in treatment to have objective confirmation of the symptoms.

A woman with vaginismus will usually be quite distressed about these involuntary spasms, over which she perceives herself to have no control. The sense of embarrassment and frustration may be enhanced if the woman remains sexually responsive, which is likely. For example, Duddle (1977) reported on 30 women seeking treatment for vaginismus. Of these, 56% were orgasmic during petting, 41% in dreams, and 28% through masturbation. Simply providing information of this nature can be therapeutic. Because there remain many myths regarding sexuality, it is possible that patients develop what might appear to professionals as curious explanations for the disorder, and that they (and their partners) may be quite self-critical. We have observed that in the absence of opportunities to talk openly with an expert, people commonly develop self-critical beliefs about their experience. These "secondary" complications often require attention in therapy.

A recent comprehensive review of the literature raises the question as to whether it is even useful to conceptualize vaginismus as a distinct syndrome (Reissing, Binik, & Khalifé, 1999). Even though the prototypical symptom of vaginismus is the involuntary spasm of the musculature of the outer third of the vagina (American Psychiatric Association, 2000), Reissing et al. (1999) point out that there is only one published study that has measured such spasms with physiological recordings, and these investigators found no differences in vaginismic women compared to controls! Reissing et al. argue further that very little has changed in our conceptualization and treatment of vaginismus since the term was first coined by Sims in 1861. These authors point out that vaginismus tends to be viewed as either a medical problem that is provoked by hypersensitivity specific to the genital organs or as a phobic (psychological) reaction resulting from fear of pain. These dual conceptualizations still exist, but the authors point out the lack of empirical support to justify their existence. Clearly, continued research regarding the fundamental nature of vaginismus is necessary.

Prevalence

There have been few broad-based epidemiological surveys regarding the prevalence of vaginismus in the general population. In two recent studies that we located, population-based estimates of vaginismus were 1% or less (Fugl-Meyer & Sjogren Fugl-Meyer, 1999; Ventegodt, 1998).

Estimates of the prevalence of vaginismus in sexual dysfunction clinics have ranged from 5% to 42% of the patients presenting for sex therapy (Bancroft & Coles, 1976; Hawton, 1982; Masters & Johnson, 1970; O'Sullivan, 1979; Renshaw, 1988). The lowest estimate comes from Renshaw (1988), but her criteria were the most stringent; that is, in her estimate, she counted only women who complained solely of vaginismus. Women with other, concurrent (i.e., comorbid) disorders (e.g., orgasmic dysfunction) were counted separately. Thus, Renshaw's estimate may be artificially low. The highest estimate comes from O'Sullivan (1979) in Ireland, and may be the product of factors unique to the Irish culture (discussed later). Finally, data from these reports probably underestimate the prevalence of vaginismus; many women with vaginismus initially seek help through fertility clinics, because vaginismus is believed to be a leading cause of the nonconsummation of marriage (see Barnes, 1981; Hawton, 1985). Thus, on the basis of data from clinic samples, it would appear that vaginismus is not an uncommon disorder.

More recent data are available from other health care settings. For example, Goldmeier et al. (1997) reported a current prevalence of 25% in a STD clinic, whereas Read et al. (1997) reported a current estimate of 30% in a primary care setting. Clinic samples indicate that there may be important differences in the prevalence of vaginismus across cultures. In Iran, Shokrollahi et al. (1999) reported that 8% of a sample of 300 healthy young, married women reported vaginismus. Barnes (1986a, 1986b) believes that lifelong vaginismus is an extremely rare clinical entity in North America and in most of western Europe, but that it is not uncommon in Ireland, eastern Europe, and Latin America. He has conducted research with Irish women and suggests that vaginismus is the most common cause of unconsummated marriages (Barnes, 1981, 1986a, 1986b). On the basis of data obtained from infertility studies, Barnes (1981) suggests that vaginismus occurs in 5 out of every 1,000 women, a rate of 0.5%. The unusually high prevalence of vaginismus among Irish women has also been reported by O'Sullivan (1979).

Etiology

BIOLOGICAL FACTORS

A number of biological causes or processes have been associated with vaginismus, and these need to be carefully evaluated in every case. In a study of 76 patients with vaginismus, Lamont (1978) found evidence for contributing physical factors in 24 patients. These factors included previous surgery (e.g., vaginal hysterectomies), episiotomy, atrophic vaginitis, *Monilia* vaginitis, *Trichomonas* vaginitis, constipation, retroversion, and pelvic congestion. Tollison and Adams (1979) have suggested that the following physical factors must be ruled out: endometriosis, relaxation of the supporting uterine ligaments, rigid hymen, hemorrhoids, painful hymenal tags, stenosis of the vagina, pelvic tumors, pelvic inflammatory disease, senile atrophy of the vagina, childbirth pathologies, and urethral caruncle. As both Lamont (1978) and Tollison and Adams (1979) point out, although most of these conditions may not be directly responsible for the vaginismus, they may be associated with vaginismus indirectly through a classical conditioning process.

PSYCHOSOCIAL FACTORS

The classical conditioning formulation of vaginismus suggests that a woman may experience significant pain (i.e., dyspareunia) upon her initial attempts at intercourse. This pain, which functions as an unconditioned stimulus, leads to a natural, self-protective tightening of the vaginal muscles (the unconditioned response). Over time, stimuli associated with vaginal penetration (e.g., the presence of one's partner without clothes) or even the thought of intercourse can become conditioned stimuli and lead to reflexive muscle spasms (the conditioned response). This classical conditioning mechanism, depicted in Figure 5.1, is strengthened by basic operant conditioning; that is, in order to prevent these spasms, a woman tries to avoid coitus; this avoidance behavior relieves her anticipatory anxiety and serves to reinforce her avoidance.

As with dyspareunia, avoidance behavior may be more likely in couples in which the male partner is particularly unassertive and overly accommodating. This is not to say that women with vaginismus should be treated more forcefully. Rather, the point we wish to make is that couples in which the male is more traditionally gender-typed are less likely to present for the treatment of vaginismus (see Case 4 in Chapter 9).

Not all instances of vaginismus, however, are classically conditioned, and a plethora of other psychosocial causes have been suggested. For example, on the basis of their experience with 19 cases of vaginismus, Masters and Johnson (1970) suggested that all of the following might be implicated: the inhibiting influence of religious orthodoxy, response to a partner's sexual dysfunction, a prior sexual trauma, and response to a sexual-orientation concern. Poinsard (1968) suggests that other factors—such as an unwillingness to assume the adult role, as well as fears of pregnancy, sexually transmitted disease, or injury—may be implicated; however, we have found little empirical support for this hypothesis.

Generally, there is limited empirical research to inform our discussion of etiology. In a rare empirical study with a comparison group, Barnes (1986b)

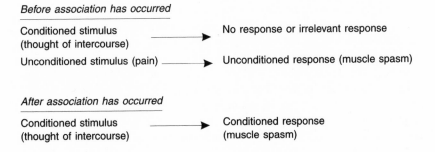

FIGURE 5.1. Classical conditioning model of vaginismus.

interviewed 53 women who presented for treatment of lifelong vaginismus. All were seen at a psychosexual clinic in Dublin, Ireland. These women were compared to 66 women treated at the same clinic for a variety of other sexual difficulties and dysfunctions (e.g., orgasmic dysfunction). The primary focus of the interview was on patients' prior relationship with their parents. Patients with vaginismus were more likely than were patients with other sexual dysfunctions to have a tyrannical father (23% vs. 9%, respectively). (Interestingly, O'Sullivan, 1979, also reported that 70% of the 23 vaginismic women he treated remembered their fathers as threatening, fearful, and often violent figures.) In addition, negative sexual conditioning that involved religious themes was more common in the vaginismic women (19% vs. 3%), as was the presence of additional psychopathology (11% vs. 1%). Surprisingly, the lifelong prevalence of sexual trauma in subjects in this study was lower than might be predicted (only 2 of 119 patients).

Tugrul and Kabakci (1997) provided additional evidence for the etiology of vaginismus. They studied the roles of family of origin, husband characteristics, anxiety, body image, and gender-role identity in 40 married Turkish women (ages 19–35 years) and their husbands who sought treatment. They found that women did not have sexual contact frequently, were not very sensual during the sexual interaction, and had fears of pain, physical harm or even death during intercourse. Trait anxiety level, wives' evaluations of their husbands as undependable, and authoritarian–oppressive attitudes of the parents were predictive of vaginismus.

Findings such as these have led Ng (1999) to suggest that vaginismus should be considered a culture-bound syndrome, with the emphasis placed on fear or resistance to vaginal penetration rather than on pain or distress as the core symptom. We need to emphasize that findings and theoretical formulations such as these, although interesting, should be considered preliminary because they are based on very small samples; additional research is clearly necessary. Indeed, recent reviews of the etiology of vaginismus (Reissing et al., 1999) point to the lack of consensus. Given the relatively impoverished knowledge base for this disorder, assessment and treatment will require creativity as well as careful treatment monitoring.

Part II

ASSESSMENT AND TREATMENT

In Chapters 2–5, we described the sexual dysfunctions and provided information on their prevalence and etiology. Now that you have an understanding of the sexual dysfunctions, we turn our attention to the practical tasks of assessment and treatment. In Chapter 6, we present a guide to the biopsychosocial assessment of the sexual dysfunctions. Although we emphasize the interview as the cornerstone of the assessment process, we also discuss the use of self-report questionnaires, as well as the use of psychophysiological and biomedical assessment. In Chapters 7 and 8, we provide the fundamentals of sex therapy as well as guidelines regarding the integration of psychosocial and biomedical approaches to the treatment of the sexual dysfunctions. Chapter 9 provides detailed assessment and treatment information for several illustrative clinical cases, and Chapter 10 concludes our presentation by discussing professional issues, such as obtaining further training and establishing a sex therapy practice.

6

Assessment

The purpose of this chapter is to provide a guide to the assessment of the sexual dysfunctions. In this chapter, we assume that you are the primary treatment provider (in Chapter 8, we supply information for situations in which you might serve as a consultant), and provide information on the use of interviewing, self-report questionnaires, and psychophysiological procedures. We also discuss how to integrate your psychosocial evaluation with data from a medical evaluation. Results from your assessment should allow you to describe the problem, formulate a working hypothesis of its etiology (i.e., predisposing, precipitating, and maintaining factors), develop an intervention plan that will target the key causal factors, provide feedback to the patient, and establish baseline functioning from which to evaluate the efficacy of treatment.

Overview of Assessment

Comprehensive and accurate assessment is crucial to formulating a helpful treatment program. A comprehensive assessment includes medical, psychosocial, and psychophysiological evaluations. We recommend that both clinical interviews and self-report questionnaires be used for the psychosocial evaluation and the evaluation process be conducted over three sessions. Regarding clinical interviews, experience teaches that obtaining meaningful information is a skill that involves far more than just asking the right questions. Assessment can be especially challenging because most people are uncomfortable discussing their sexual behaviors. Our patients are often nervous about discussing their sexual concerns; they need to feel relaxed and supported. Furthermore, many individuals may have strong beliefs about what sexual conduct is acceptable or unacceptable, and they may be offended if a therapist's views do not agree with their own.

Assessment should begin with an appropriate introduction for the patient(s). During this time, the assessment structure and content should be outlined. We prefer to do this while both partners are present. We might begin by saying:

> "Today, in this first interview, I would like to obtain some background information and get an understanding of what brought you here today. I find it helpful to begin by talking to a couple together for a little while to answer questions, but then I would like to be able to spend time with each of you separately. Thus, in this session I will talk to one of you alone; then, in our next session, I will talk to the other person. It doesn't matter whom I start with. It is up to you, but it may be best to start with whomever has the busiest schedule. While I am talking to one of you, the other person can fill out some questionnaires.
>
> "After we have met and talked individually, I may suggest that you undergo a medical examination so that we have all the information we need to make progress most efficiently.
>
> "On our third meeting, we can all meet together and I will review my thoughts about your situation. At this time, I will try to explain what I believe to be the factors that originally caused your difficulty, as well as any factors that may be maintaining it. If appropriate, I will outline a treatment plan, targeted toward the important factors, to help you. So that is what the process is like. I imagine that we could complete this within 1–2 weeks. Do you have any questions or issues you would like to discuss before we break up and I talk to one of you?"

As the therapist, you should also mention your credentials and let the couple know that you are comfortable dealing with sexual problems. You should convey to the couple that overcoming sexual difficulties requires the cooperative efforts of both partners. This is necessary to address because such a couple often believes that (1) one person is to blame for the problems, and (2) it is the role of the therapist to identify and "cure" the "guilty/sick" one. After you have said this, however, it is important to interview each person separately, following the introduction, to gather accurate information that is unencumbered by a partner's presence. Time can be wasted if the partners are always seen together. Many individuals have hidden stories (e.g., affairs, homosexual interests) that would never be revealed in the presence of their partners; yet this information is vital for developing a case formulation and planning the therapy program.

After the introductory remarks, the partners should be invited to ask any questions they might have. The remainder of the first session is then spent interviewing one of the partners alone. The other partner is asked to complete a set of self-report questionnaires during this time. We sometimes allow patients to take questionnaires home and complete them there, especially if time constraints prevent them from completing the questionnaires in the office. However, we ask that they complete them independently, and that the partners do not share the questionnaires.

The second session is used to interview the other partner alone, while the person interviewed during the first session completes his or her questionnaires. The third session can be used to assess the interaction of the couple. During this session, you can observe how the partners communicate and interact with each other. Problems and strengths in communication readily emerge at this time—for example, you can assess how caring, hostile, honest, and so on, the couple appears to be. It is also important to determine how much trust each partner has in the other; we try to do this by comparing the amount of self-disclosure that occurs during the couple session with that in the earlier individual sessions. This third session is also designated to present an initial case formulation and provide an outline of the therapy plan.

In our work, we find that skillful interviewing serves as the cornerstone of the assessment process. Of course, this view is not unique to the domain of the sexual dysfunctions. Indeed, many fine articles, chapters, and books have been written on skillful interviewing (e.g., Morganstern, 1988; Pope, 1979, Turkat, 1986). We recommend that you study these works for the general information and insights they provide about interviewing. In this chapter, however, we focus our discussion on the issues that pertain specifically to interviewing patients about sexual problems.

Despite its importance, not all health professionals know how to react to a patient's sexual concerns. We have had numerous patients report to us that they have tried previously to discuss their sexual problems with their physicians or therapists but were met with embarrassment or lack of interest; as a result, the patients did not pursue their concerns. For example, a 70-year-old female patient told us that she tried to discuss her vaginal dryness problem with her physician. Unfortunately for our patient, the physician avoided further discussion of this problem and only later referred to it as her "other problem." She sensed his discomfort with the subject and did not raise the problem again. She later told us, "You know, my doctor was too embarrassed to even say the word 'sex,' so he made me feel weird for asking about it."

A recent study by Read, King, and Watson (1997) provides additional evidence that sexual dysfunctions are often neglected by primary care physicians. Using a survey of patients in a primary care setting, they learned that 70% of the patients considered sexual matters to be an appropriate topic to discuss with their doctor. Thirty-five percent of the men and 42% of the women acknowledged a sexual dysfunction in the survey. Despite patients recognizing the importance of sexual problems and revealing specific concerns, a later chart review indicated that sexual problems were recorded in only 2% of the practitioners' notes.

Another, more damaging example of physician's inappropriate reaction to their patient's sexual concerns has been when advice is given without a thorough assessment. We have encountered several cases in which male patients have been told by their physicians to seek out other sexual partners if they were having trouble functioning with their wives. The possibility of creating additional sexual problems, as well as potential relationship and even possible legal problems, was seemingly never considered.

Despite these risks, research indicates that self-disclosure, at least in moderation, is associated with improved mental health and relationship outcomes (Cozby, 1973); in general, women tend to self-disclose more than do men. However, both men and women find it difficult to disclose sexual feelings, fantasies, and fears. Several investigators have reported that when asked to indicate the secrets that would be most threatening to disclose, individuals typically identify sexually related material as the most risky (e.g., Norton, Feldman, & Tafoya, 1974); this is especially true for women (e.g., Solano, 1981).

Thus, when we ask patients to disclose information about their sexual lives, it is important to keep in mind that we are asking them to disclose their deepest (and for some, their darkest) secrets (Norton et al., 1974). Chances are good that they may not have disclosed this material to anyone, including their spouse or their closest confidante. The disclosure holds much promise for self- and relationship-related development and growth, but it remains quite risky for our patients.

Moreover, in a time when our popular culture is awash with sexual messages and communication—music videos, AIDS prevention messages, internet chat sites, advertisements for products such as Viagra—sexual concerns have increasingly been normalized and legitimized. This trend in popular culture has resulted in a greater likelihood that patients will bring forth sexual complaints to physicians and health care practitioners. Thus, it is important that all professional health care practitioners be skillful at handling these concerns and not create additional problems.

Step-by-Step Details of Interviewing: Sessions 1 and 2

We begin by proposing that an interview will best serve the needs of the patient if you obtain important information in a sensitive and efficient manner.

Toward this end, we believe that the crucial components of an effective clinical interview include (1) making assumptions (hypotheses) before the interview; (2) setting goals for the interview; (3) attending to process throughout the interview; and (4) following a specific structure and content during the interview.

Assumptions

Assumptions are the hypotheses that a clinician makes in order to gather the most accurate information without wasting time and effort. Assumptions reflect the preferred direction of error. Thus, for example, it is better at the beginning to assume a low level of verbal understanding on the part of a patient and thus to direct language to the patient in a clear and concrete manner. Obviously, as a clinician learns more about a patient, these assumptions are adjusted.

Other examples of useful assumptions include the following:

- Clients will be embarrassed and have difficulty discussing sexual matters.
- Clients will not understand medically correct terminology.
- Clients will be misinformed about sexual functioning.
- Clients will be in crisis and may be suicidal.
- Clients have not been open with each other and do not freely discuss sexual matters.

As an example of a common misunderstanding, we can report the following. It is not unusual for men to misunderstand the occurrence of a nocturnal erection. Many will misattribute this response to having a full bladder. This misattribution undoubtedly developed because when men wake up at night to urinate, they often have erections, followed by detumescence as the man begins to "wake up." We have heard physicians speak of "full-bladder erections," showing that this misunderstanding is widespread and not confined to less educated people. It is interesting that most men do not see an inconsistency in their logic, based on lack of erection during the daytime when they have to urinate.

Goals

Goals are the desired outcomes established before each session to give the assessment procedure a focus. At times, the goals have to be adjusted as information is learned to accommodate the needs of the patient. However, adhering closely to the goals will help make the therapy more efficient by helping to minimize sidetracking.

Examples of the goals you might set for the first session include the following:

- Establish rapport.
- Obtain a general description of sexual problems.
- Obtain a thorough psychosocial history.
- Obtain a description of other life concerns and current stressors.
- Determine whether sex therapy is appropriate for the patient/couple at this time.

With regard to the last-mentioned goal, there are no specific guidelines for making this determination. Thus, a therapist should determine on a case-by-case basis whether working on a sexual problem will benefit a patient/couple. Certainly, if either partner is depressed and/or overly anxious, or if there is a great deal of anger, then it is more appropriate to address nonsexual issues first. In some cases, sexual difficulties may be insignificant in light of other problems. Furthermore, effective assessment and therapy require collaboration between both partners and the therapist that is compromised in the presence of such hostility. Similarly, there may be very dysfunctional communication between partners that must be addressed before sexual issues can be effectively confronted.

Process

"Process" is the term that describes the interaction between a patient and a therapist; this interaction can either facilitate or inhibit the assessment. When we use the term "process," we also mean to include the physical setting (Is it private? professional?), the therapist's appearance (competent, trustworthy) and presentation (well-prepared, informed, calm, friendly, accepting), as well as the more common meanings of the term "process." It is clear that many clinicians feel uncomfortable dealing with sexual problems. Personal feelings of shock and embarrassment will often show through attempts to be friendly and accepting. Mismanagement of these negative feelings could be divisive and create a barrier to effective therapy. If a therapist's feelings cannot be managed appropriately, then he or she should not be dealing with sexual problems. Patients readily discern embarrassment or incompetence—as did the patients we mentioned earlier.

Additional examples of process factors that can sabotage assessment (and subsequent therapy as well) include differences between the therapist and patients in terms of age, gender, and/or ethnicity; and erotic attractions or interpersonal repulsions between therapist and patient. With the exception of erotic attractions, other factors between therapist and patient should be addressed openly in the assessment process. For example, a young male therapist may wish to address gender and age differences in the assessment of an elderly woman presenting with decreased sexual desire following onset of menopause. This may be approached as follows:

"Mrs. Jones, you are here to discuss and obtain help for a sexual problem and I am wondering if talking to a young male therapist about such matters makes you uncomfortable or even inhibited to do so? Talking about sexual matters to any stranger is often difficult for most people but I wonder if you feel you may have a problem talking to me."

By presenting this issue for discussion, you acknowledge (and give the patient permission to express) a normal amount of discomfort or embarrassment regarding the discussion of sexual material. Also, you will ask the patient to express honestly whether his or her anxiety may interfere with the assessment or therapy process. Finally, by raising the topics of age and gender, you will have presented yourself as a sensitive and understanding therapist. If a patient expresses an unacceptable level of discomfort, then you should make every effort to refer the patient to a therapist whose characteristics may better serve him or her.

There may be other circumstances that require a referral to serve the patient best, for example, if you lack the technical expertise or the life experience to help a particular patient. As we discuss later, some clinicians may not feel comfortable or prepared to work with gay, lesbian, or bisexual patients. Alternatively, a younger therapist may not be able to appreciate fully the challenges faced by a widow as she tries to overcome continued attachment to her first husband while she attempts to build a relationship with a new partner. And, from time to time, gender matching of patient and therapist may be most appropriate. Under such circumstances, the ethically responsible decision is to refer the patient to a therapist who is better suited to his or her needs.

Finally, in some instances, you may have a strong attraction (or negative feelings) toward a patient. In such cases, we advise against disclosing your feelings to the patient; rather, refer him or her to another therapist. Each of us as therapists may have our own style in handling such situations, but, generally, you should tell the patient that you feel another therapist could better serve him or her.

Structure and Content

"Structure" and "content" refer to the ordering of questions to be asked, and the areas to be covered, respectively. In general, it is to the patient's benefit for a therapist to get to the heart of the patient's concerns. Thus, spending several sessions "breaking the ice" or "establishing a relationship" is not warranted in most cases. (An exception to this general rule occurs when prior intimate or therapeutic relationships have been quite unstable; in such cases, it may be necessary to devote several sessions to establishing trust.) In all instances, it is useful to get a general sense of the patient's history, especially as it relates to his or her sexual adjustment.

The outline provided here is meant solely as a guide. This suggested order should not be followed blindly but should be modified depending upon the clinical circumstances. We do not advise following an invariant order of questions for all patients. Instead, the structure and content of the interview should reflect the needs of the patient. There are frequently crisis issues to which you must attend before sexual matters can be addressed. Or it may be important to allow a patient to digress beyond the usual structure, but only if the digression contributes ultimately to a better understanding of the patient or his or her problem.

With this recognition of the need to individualize the interview structure and content for each patient, we nevertheless suggest the following order that might be a useful beginning or "default" structure for your use:

1. Start with nonthreatening demographics (e.g., age, marital status, who lives in household, current employment, educational background, address, telephone number).

2. Continue with the open-ended question "What brings you here today?" Notice how freely and comfortably the patient discusses sexual matters in general, and his or her particular difficulty. Use probes and directive comments to keep the patient's report on target. Once you reach a general impression concerning the scope of the sexual problem, then move on to the detailed chronological history.

3. Obtain a psychosexual and psychosocial history.

a. *Childhood*. Ask about the family structure and experiences when the patient was a child. Also ask about social status, abuse or neglect, first sexual experience (upsetting or pleasant?), parents' relationship, alcohol and substance abuse, messages about sex, and any other information that emerges as potentially relevant.

When asking about sexual abuse or trauma, we encourage you to follow the recommendation of Becker (1989), an expert in this area, who recommends that you ask patients whether they have ever been the recipients of *unwanted* sexual acts. Use of the word "unwanted" allows patients to report experiences that they might not reveal if asked about "rape" or "abuse." In this regard, mention that many women are reluctant to identify sexual violations committed by boyfriends, husbands, and others who are known to them. We also wish to alert you to the potential importance of vicarious trauma experiences.

As reviewed in earlier chapters, it is now understood that Child Sexual Abuse (CSA) is a powerful cause of many adult disorders (Beitchman et al., 1992). Thus, we wish to stress the importance of assessing this history.

b. *Adolescence.* Inquire about relationships with peers, self-esteem and body image, dating, sexual experiences (both homosexual and heterosexual), menarche in females, success–failure in school, substance use, and any other information that emerges as potentially relevant. Check again for unwanted sexual experiences.

c. *Adult.* Ask about significant relationships and events after age 20; try to address self-esteem, marriage/relationship history, sexual experiences, and so forth. Check again for unwanted sexual experiences. Inquire about any unusual sexual experiences, as well as psychiatric history or treatment.

d. *Current sexual functioning.* Acquire details regarding sexual and nonsexual experiences in the current relationship, recent changes in sexual functioning and/or satisfaction, flexibility in sexual attitudes and behaviors, extramarital affairs, strengths and weaknesses of the partner, likes and dislikes regarding the partner's sexual behavior, and so on.

4. Obtain a brief medical history.

a. Ask about significant childhood/teenage diseases, surgery, medical care, congenital disorders, and the like. Ask men and women about how they experienced secondary sex changes (particularly menarche, in the case of women).

b. Pay particular attention to the medical history after age 20; ask about any significant diseases, surgery, medical care, and so forth. Be sure to ask about the following: Has the patient received regular medical care? (If not, refer to medical workup.) Is the patient currently taking prescribed medication? Is the patient currently being treated for any medical problems? Ask women about menstrual difficulties and, if appropriate, menopause.

c. A critically important task is to assess both partners in a couple for history of sexually transmitted diseases (STDs). During the past two decades, we have witnessed an unprecedented pandemic of STDs, especially HIV. Worldwide, estimates suggest that 10 million people have acquired immunodeficiency syndrome, or AIDS, with another 30 million persons infected with HIV (Carey, 1999). Other STDs are even more prevalent. For example, genital herpes currently affects 40 million U.S. citizens, with an additional 500,000 cases occurring annually. Chlamydia affects approximately 4 million U.S. citizens and is known to be the most common bacterial-like STD infection. Such data require that sex therapists inquire about STD history and current status, and help their patients to avoid future infection. Anyone who is sexually active is at risk, regardless of sexual orientation, drug use, or medical history. You should ask each partner in a dyad separately about history of STDs and testing for HIV. If the couple's history together is recent, or includes other partners, and if both partners have not been tested recently for HIV, it is wise to suggest that they use condoms during insertive sexual behavior until HIV testing has been completed. We advise this as a standard precaution to protect your patients against infection.

5. Be sensitive to potential covert issues. Ask whether there are any issues that the patient does not want discussed in front of his or her partner. What significant conflict exists (impressions of one's partner or hidden experiences)? *We believe strongly in creating an interview environment in which each partner can be assured of confidentiality.* Without separate confidential interviews, crucial information may remain hidden. For example, consider the case of Mr. and Mrs. W.

Mr. and Mrs. Williams, ages 56 and 54, respectively, had been married 26 years; they had two college-age daughters. Both Mr. and Mrs. Williams were professionals with graduate degrees. At the first session, they both agreed that the problem was Mr. Williams's lack of sexual desire. In fact, the couple had not had sexual relations for about 10 years. Mrs. Williams was clearly very angry, although both partners expressed a desire to stay in the marriage. Following a discussion of the assessment structure and therapy process, Mr. Williams asked to stay for his individual assessment session while Mrs. Williams retired to the waiting room.

Mr. Williams expressed great relief at being able to talk to the therapist alone, confidentially. He revealed in this session that he had been using male homosexual magazines as a masturbatory outlet for a number of years. More recently, he had started visiting homosexual websites on the internet. At the point of the assessment interview, he had denied any actual sexual contact with males, although he had thought of it often.

Mr. Williams was not prepared to share the information about homosexuality with his wife because he felt for sure she would immediately leave the marriage. He also felt that his interest in homosexual stimulation was not a causative factor, because his lack of sexual interest in his wife began years before his interest in male homosexual erotica.

Obviously, this was a complicated case with many delicate issues. The important point of this case is that had separate interviews not been held, the therapist would never have known about the very important issue of Mr. Williams's use of erotic materials. Knowing this information was essential for developing an overall treatment strategy. This couple, and all couples, are also told at the onset that it may be best to deal with either person alone at times in order to work through specific issues. As it turned out, therapy did begin with individual therapy for Mr. Williams.

There are some issues that, although raised in individual meetings, must—ultimately—be addressed conjointly. An extreme example might be an instance where one partner confides that he or she has a viral STD about which his or her partner does not know. Here, we would work with the infected partner to help him or her determine how best to share this information. This disclosure will often need to be done in session, and its meaning for the relationship will need to be processed. There is also the need to plan for treatment of the infected partner, and prevention of new infections in both partners.

In most cases, the infected partner agrees that such disclosure is appropriate but has been afraid (or not sure how) to do this. This is where you can be very helpful, using problem solving, role plays, and rehearsal in individual meetings (Kalichman, 1998). If the infected person refuses to share this information with his or her partner, then you face an ethical dilemma. On the one hand, you have an obligation to honor the confidence of the infected person; on the other hand, you have the duty to warn the partner against the possibility of infection (Knapp & VandeCreek, 1990; Melchert & Patterson, 1999; Zonana, 1989). Because of the complex and evolving legal and ethical opinions regarding your responsibilities under such circumstances, we advise you to consult with your State Health Department, professional colleagues, and organizations regarding the best way to resolve such a dilemma should it arise in an assessment. The circumstances surrounding such rare cases are unique and must be considered thoroughly.

6. Provide each patient with a second opportunity to reveal anything he or she thinks may be relevant. In this regard, LoPiccolo and Heiman (1978) recommend ending the interview by asking, "Is there anything else that you would like to tell me about your background that you feel bears on your sexual life?"

The second interview is with the other partner. We ask this partner whether anything has changed since the first interview, and whether the partner has discussed the first interview with him or her. The answers to these queries will yield information about a couple's interaction pattern, openness in communication, and ability to schedule time for important issues. It is also important to ask this partner whether there are any issues or questions that he or she would like addressed before the interview begins. This open-ended approach allows the discussion of process issues (such as a patient's doubt about a therapist's qualifications) as well as important personal issues that may have an impact on the therapy (such as a patient's affair or a death in the family).

Once the open-ended issues are dealt with, then you may move on to the interview proper, following the structure and content outline for the first interview.

Self-Report Questionnaires: Sessions 1 and 2

During each partner's initial interview with the therapist, the other partner is asked to complete a number of self-report questionnaires. Self-report questionnaires are standardized, easily administered and scored instruments that can be filled out by the patient in a relatively short period and provide additional information about a patient's situation at any point in time and/or over a period of many administrations (Fisher & Corcoran, 1994a, 1994b). These questionnaires have many potential advantages. First, because they provide extensive information at little cost, they are cost-effective. Second, they allow a patient to organize his or her thoughts in a reflective, considered way that is not always possible within the time constraints of an interview. Third, self-report questionnaires permit patients to disclose sensitive information that they might not reveal or might find difficult to verbalize during a "live" interaction. Fourth, they allow you to assess a patient's progress over time, making treatment evaluation more precise and less prone to therapist-related biases. Fifth, self-report questionnaires allow you to compare your patient to other individuals (with the help of established norms); thus, in difficult diagnostic cases, these questionnaires can provide a known metric against which to make judgments. Sixth, the questionnaires can serve as an additional stimulus that encourages a patient to think through aspects of his or her sexuality. Seventh, if used after the interview, self-report questionnaires help you to evaluate the validity of a diagnostic or etiological formulation (see Carey et al., 1984). Alternatively, if used before the interview, self-report measures can serve as screening devices that help you as the interviewer to be more efficient in getting to the heart of the presenting complaint.

We do not recommend that you use a standard "battery" of measures for every patient/couple. Instead, we recommend that you select questionnaires that are likely to yield the most helpful information.

Locating Questionnaires on Your Own

Obtaining good questionnaires has been difficult in the past. Many research-oriented journals that provided psychometric information (e.g., reliability, validity) on new measures did not publish the actual questionnaires. Clinical sources that provided the items often did not provide psychometric characteristics. As a result, many practitioners have resorted to homemade instruments of dubious quality. Fortunately, it is now easier to learn about and obtain self-report questionnaires for clinical use.

Professional journals provide an outlet for authors who wish to make their questionnaires available to other users. These journals are available at most university and medical center libraries, or they can be ordered from professional organizations. Professional journals are increasingly available online (sometimes for free, sometimes for a fee). Also available online are search engines such as Medline and PsychLit that make it easier to find information quickly. Medline can be searched for free from the National Library of Medicine website (*www.nlm.nih.gov*) whereas PsychLit is a pay service available from the American Psychological Association (*www.apa.org*). General search engines such as AltaVista (*www.altavista.com*), Yahoo (*www.yahoo.com*), and Google (*www.google.com*) can also yield questionnaires that are actually posted online and can be downloaded for your use. However, such searches typically do not control for quality, and we advise that you select measures that have been demonstrated to be reliable and valid before using them with patients.

If electronic searching seems like too much trouble, or if you want a ready supply of measures at your fingertips, there are also books devoted to the use of self-report questionnaires. For general mental health measures, we have found Fisher and Corcoran's (1994a, 1994b) two books, *Measures for Clinical Practice: A Sourcebook*, to be quite useful. (Volume 1 is devoted to measures for couples, families, and children, whereas volume 2 is devoted to adults. Thus, unfortunately, it may be necessary to purchase both books if you desire measures for both adults and couples.) For measures related to physical health and adjustment, we recommend McDowell and Newell's (1996) *Measuring Health: A Guide to Rating Scales and Questionnaires*. Finally, for measures of sexual functioning, we recommend Davis, Yarber, Bauserman, Schneer, and Davis's (1998) book, *Handbook of Sexually-Related Measures*, a treasure trove that warrants your attention. All three of these references are second editions, which reflects their usefulness. We expect that books such as this will continue to be updated in the coming years, because they are quite useful.

Once you learn of a questionnaire, you will want to evaluate it along several important dimensions.

1. *Psychometric strength.* Is it reliable (i.e., individual items consistent with one another, scores stable over time) and valid (i.e., it measures what it purports to measure, rather than measuring some other construct, such as intelligence or social desirability)? These criteria may seem overly technical, but we encourage you not to overlook them. A measure that is not reliable and/or valid is not only worthless, but it could also distort your understanding of your patient.

2. *Clinical relevance.* Does the measure address the clinical issues at hand? For example, if you are concerned primarily with evaluating a patient's level of sexual desire, it would not be fruitful to ask him or her to complete the Minnesota Multiphasic Personality Inventory (MMPI; a global personality measure), or even the Sexual Opinion Survey (SOS), because these instruments provide no information on desire. Also, it is true that

many instruments are not intended for clinical use and have little or no clinical utility; however, there are also a large number of well-conceived and useful measures. You need to determine the clinical relevance for each measure you use with each patient on a case-by-case basis.

3. *Practicality or feasibility.* Is the questionnaire at a reading and vocabulary level appropriate for your patients? We have found that many questionnaires use vocabulary that is beyond most patients. One source for information on reading levels of a variety of older sexually-relevant questionnaires is a paper by Jensen, Witcher, and Upton (1987). Although this paper has not, to our knowledge, been updated, there now exists user-friendly computer software that can assess reading level on most personal computers (e.g., word processing software).

4. *Comparability.* Are there normative data against which to compare your patient's scores? Here, you will need to be sure that the normative sample is appropriate for your patients. Thus, if a questionnaire was normed with males ages 50–70 years and your patients tend to be young females, the normative data are probably not useful. Also, be aware that many questionnaires have been normed on college students and may not be representative of your patients.

5. *Cost.* Does the measure cost you or your patient too much time and/ or money to use? Some instruments (e.g., the MMPI) are so long that many patients find them annoying and, as a result, do not respond in a cooperative fashion. Other measures are expensive to obtain and/or administer. You should know, however, that many measures are in the public domain and can be used for free.

Given these criteria, we have identified several worthwhile measures that you may want to consider for use in your work. We have found them useful in our own work and describe them next. Actual copies of several of these measures can be found at the end of this chapter.

Specific Self-Report Questionnaires

MEDICAL HISTORY FORM (SEE TABLE 6.1)

As indicated in earlier chapters, it is necessary that we be well informed about the health history of our patients. Knowledge of ailments such as diabetes and cardiovascular disease that can have a direct pathophysiological effect on sexual functioning should be obtained on each male and female patient. Equally important is information on past or present medical conditions that may indirectly impact on sexual functioning. It is important for the clinician to assess any medical condition that causes pain or discomfort or effects self-confidence or self-image. It is these indirect medical conditions that are most

TABLE 6.1. Medical History Form

Past medical history

Please circle if you have had problems with or are presently complaining of any of the following:

High blood pressure	Endometriosis	Vaginal dryness
Gall bladder	Diabetes	Pelvic inflammatory disease
Blood disorder	Blood in stool	
Arthritis	Colitis	Headache
Heart disease	Ulcers	Low back problems
Cancer	Chest pain/tightness	Pain on urination
Shortness of breath	Swollen ankles	Venereal disease
Palpitations	Lightheadedness	Difficulty urinating
Rheumatic fever	Asthma	Frequent urination
Persistent cough	TB	Kidney stones
Abdominal pain	Indigestion/heartburn	Gout
Anxiety/depression	Anemia	Neurological condition
Retinitis pigmentosa	Prostatectomy	Alcohol or drug abuse
Nausea/vomiting	Skin disease	Other: _____

Treatment history

What treatments (if any) have you received for sexual difficulties in the past? (Please circle all that apply.)

Vasodilator injections	Vaginal lubricant	Psychotherapy
Hormone therapy	MUSE	Couple/individual sex therapy
Viagra	Vacuum device	
Oral medication (other than Viagra, e.g., yohimbine)		Penile implant
		Marital/relationship counseling

Operations (include dates)

_____   _____   _____
_____   _____   _____
_____   _____   _____

Other hospitalizations

_____   _____   _____
_____   _____   _____
_____   _____   _____

(*continued on next page*)

TABLE 6.1. (*continued*)

Medications (including over-the-counter medications, vitamins, and herbal preparations)

Medication	Dose	Medication	Dose
_____	_____	_____	_____
_____	_____	_____	_____
_____	_____	_____	_____
_____	_____	_____	_____

Family history

Has anyone in your family (grandparents, parents, or siblings) ever had the following (please circle all that apply):

Illness	Relationship	Age when diagnosed
Cancer (type): _____	_____	_____
Hypertension	_____	_____
Heart disease	_____	_____
Diabetes	_____	_____
Stroke	_____	_____
Mental disease	_____	_____
Drug or alcohol addiction	_____	_____
Glaucoma	_____	_____
Blood disease	_____	_____
Other: _____	_____	_____

General medical

Do you use tobacco? _____ Yes _____ No

If yes, in what form? _____ In what amount? (e.g., packs per day) _____

Do you drink alcohol? _____ Yes _____ No
If yes, how much per week? _____

Do you drink coffee/tea? _____ Yes _____ No
If yes, how much per week? _____

Do you use drugs such as marijuana or cocaine? _____ Yes _____ No
If yes, please state drug and how often it is used: _____

How you ever engaged in any activity that would put you at risk of contracting AIDS? _____ Yes _____ No
If yes, please explain: _____

often overlooked by both patients and clinicians when trying to sort out all of the factors contributing to sexual dysfunction. We have found the medical history form presented in the Table 6.1 as a useful tool to gather important medical information for use in sex therapy. Obviously, this form is not meant to be used for medical diagnosis and no medical advice should ever be given to a patient by a nonphysician. The form is meant as a guide to consider possible contributions to interference with sexual functioning. If this form does not serve you well, you might study forms used by health maintenance organizations or other medical practices, or simply develop one of your own to guide your assessment.

BRIEF INDEX OF SEXUAL FUNCTIONING FOR WOMEN
(BISF-W; SEE TABLE 6.2)

The BISF-W (Taylor, Rosen, & Leiblum, 1994) is a 22-item self-report measure that assesses female sexual desire, arousal, orgasm, and sexual satisfaction. Additional items address body image, partner satisfaction, and sexual anxiety. The BISF-W can be completed in 15 minutes. The psychometric properties of the BISF-W were evaluated using a heterogeneous sample, including lesbian and bisexual women. Factor analyses have shown the BISF-W to contain three factors: sexual desire, sexual activity, and sexual satisfaction. The item relating to body image did not load on any factor, but had an eigenvalue greater than 1 and is thus scored individually. Because the internal consistency for the sexual desire factor is low ($\alpha = .39$), we prefer the Sexual Desire Inventory, described next, to assess desire. The 4-week test–retest reliability coefficients ranged from .68 to .78 for the three factors. The Derogatis Sexual Functioning Inventory (DSFI; Derogatis & Melisaratos, 1979) was used to establish concurrent validity. The results showed correlations between the three factors and their respective DSFI subtests to range from .59 to .69.

SEXUAL DESIRE INVENTORY (SDI; SEE TABLE 6.3)

The SDI (Spector, Carey, & Steinberg, 1996) assesses two dimensions of sexual desire: dyadic sexual desire (interest in behaving sexually with a partner) and solitary sexual desire (interest in behaving sexually by oneself). The SDI contains 14 items and can be completed in less than 5 minutes. Evidence of its reliability and validity is ample (Spector et al., 1996). Research with the SDI indicates that men typically have higher levels of desire than do women; use of the SDI with both partners allows the clinician to obtain a discrepancy score, which can be useful in case formulation and in providing feedback to partners. The SDI might also prove helpful in the evaluation of male orgasmic disorder; if Apfelbaum's (2000) hypotheses are correct, men with this disorder

TABLE 6.2. Brief Index of Sexual Functioning for Women (BISF-W)

Answer the following questions by choosing the most accurate response *for the past month.*

1. Do you currently have a sex partner? _____ Yes _____ No

2. Have you been sexually active during the past month? _____ Yes _____ No

3. During the past month, how frequently have you had sexual thoughts, fantasies, or erotic dreams? (Please circle the most appropriate response.)

   (0) Not at all
   (1) Once
   (2) 2 or 3 times
   (3) Once a week
   (4) 2 or 3 times per week
   (5) Once a day
   (6) More than once a day

4. Using the scale to the right, indicate how frequently you have felt a desire to engage in the following activities during the past month. (An answer is required for each, even if it may not apply to you.)

Kissing	_____	(0) Not at all
Masturbation alone	_____	(1) Once
Mutual masturbation	_____	(2) 2 or 3 times
Petting or foreplay	_____	(3) Once a week
Oral sex	_____	(4) 2 or 3 times a week
Vaginal penetration	_____	(5) Once a day
or intercourse		(6) More than once a day
Anal sex	_____	

5. Using the scale to the right, indicate how frequently you have become aroused by the following sexual experiences during the past month. (An answer is required for each, even if it may not apply to you.)

Kissing	_____	
Masturbation alone	_____	(0) Have not engaged in this activity
Mutual masturbation	_____	(1) Not at all
Petting or foreplay	_____	(2) Seldom, less than 25% of the time
Oral sex	_____	(3) Sometimes, about 50% of the time
Vaginal penetration	_____	(4) Usually, about 75% of the time
or intercourse		(5) Always became aroused
Anal sex	_____	

6. Overall, during the past month, how frequently have you become anxious or inhibited during sexual activity with a partner? (Please circle the most appropriate response.)

   (0) I have not had a partner.
   (1) Not at all anxious or inhibited

TABLE 6.2. (*continued*)

(2) Seldom, less than 25% of the time
(3) Sometimes, about 50% of the time
(4) Usually, about 75% of the time
(5) Always became anxious or inhibited

7. Using the scale to the right, indicate how frequently you have engaged in the following sexual experiences during the past month. (An answer is required for each, even if it may not apply to you.)

Kissing	____	(0) Not at all
Masturbation alone	____	(1) Once
Mutual masturbation	____	(2) 2 or 3 times
Petting or foreplay	____	(3) Once a week
Oral sex	____	(4) 2 or 3 times a week
Vaginal penetration	____	(5) Once a day
or intercourse		(6) More than once a day
Anal sex	____	

8. During the past month, who has usually initiated sexual activity? (Please circle the most appropriate response.)

   (0) I have not had a partner.
   (1) I have not had sex with a partner during the past month.
   (2) I usually have initiated activity.
   (3) My partner and I have equally initiated activity.
   (4) My partner usually has initiated activity.

9. During the past month, how have you usually responded to your partner's sexual advances? (Please circle the most appropriate response.)

   (0) I have not had a partner.
   (1) Has not happened during the past month
   (2) Usually refused
   (3) Sometimes refused
   (4) Accepted reluctantly
   (5) Accepted, but not necessarily with pleasure
   (6) Usually accepted with pleasure
   (7) Always accepted with pleasure

10. During the past month, have you felt pleasure from any form of sexual experience? (Please circle the most appropriate response.)

    (0) I have not had a partner.
    (1) Have had no sexual experience during the past month
    (2) Seldom, less than 25% of the time
    (3) Sometimes, about 50% of the time
    (4) Usually, about 75% of the time
    (5) Always felt pleasure

(*continued*)

TABLE 6.2. (*continued*)

11. Using the scale to the right, indicate how often you have reached orgasm during the past month with the following activities. (An answer is required for each, even if it may not apply to you.)

In dreams or fantasy _____
Kissing _____   (0) I have not had a partner.
Masturbation alone _____   (1) Have not engaged in this activity
Mutual masturbation _____   (2) Not at all
Petting and foreplay _____   (3) Seldom, less than 25% of the time
Oral sex _____   (4) Sometimes, about 50% of the time
Vaginal penetration _____   (5) Usually, about 75% of the time
    or intercourse   (6) Always reached orgasm
Anal sex _____

12. During the past month, has the frequency of your sexual activity with a partner been (please circle the most appropriate response):

(0) I have not had a partner
(1) Less than you desired
(2) As much as you desired
(3) More than you desired

13. Using the scale to the right, indicate the level of change, if any, in the following areas during the past month. (An answer is required for each, even if it may not apply to you.)

Sexual interest _____   (0) Not applicable
Sexual arousal _____   (1) Much lower level
Sexual activity _____   (2) Somewhat lower level
Sexual satisfaction _____   (3) No change
Sexual anxiety _____   (4) Somewhat higher level
                                        (5) Much higher level

14. During the past month, how frequently have you experienced the following? (An answer is required for each, even if it may not apply to you.)

Bleeding or irritation after vaginal
    penetration or intercourse _____   (0) Not at all
Lack of vaginal lubrication _____   (1) Seldom, less than 25%
Painful penetration or intercourse _____   of the time
Difficulty reaching orgasm _____   (2) Sometimes, about 50%
Vaginal tightness _____   of the time
Involuntary urination _____   (3) Usually, about 75%
Headaches after sexual activity _____   of the time
Vaginal infection _____   (4) Always

TABLE 6.2. (continued)

15. Using the scale to the right, indicate the frequency with which the following factors have influenced your level of sexual activity during the past month. (An answer is required for each, even if it may not apply to you.)

My own health problem
  (e.g., infection, illness)   ____
My partner's health problems   ____
Conflict in the relationship   ____
Lack of privacy   ____
Other (please specify):

_____   ____
_____   ____

(0) I have not had a partner.
(1) Not at all
(2) Seldom, less than 25%
  of the time
(3) Sometimes, about 50%
  of the time
(4) Usually, about 75%
  of the time
(5) Always

16. How satisfied are you with the overall appearance of your body? (Please circle the most appropriate response.)

(0) Very satisfied
(1) Somewhat satisfied
(2) Neither satisfied nor dissatisfied
(3) Somewhat dissatisfied
(4) Very dissatisfied

17. During the past month, how frequently have you been able to communicate your sexual desires or preferences to your partner? (Please circle the most appropriate response.)

(0) I have not had a partner
(1) I have been unable to communicate my desires or preferences
(2) Seldom, less than 25% of the time
(3) Sometimes, about 50% of the time
(4) Usually, about 75% of the time
(5) I was always able to communicate my desires and preferences

18. Overall, how satisfied have you been with your sexual relationship with your partner? (Please circle the most appropriate response.)

(0) I have not had a partner
(1) Very satisfied
(2) Somewhat satisfied
(3) Neither satisfied nor dissatisfied
(4) Somewhat dissatisfied
(5) Very dissatisfied

(continued)

TABLE 6.2. (*continued*)

19. Overall, how satisfied do you think your partner has been with your sexual relationship? (Please circle the most appropriate response.)

    (0) I have not had a partner
    (1) Very satisfied
    (2) Somewhat satisfied
    (3) Neither satisfied nor dissatisfied
    (4) Somewhat dissatisfied
    (5) Very dissatisfied

20. Overall, how important a part of your life is your sexual activity? (Please circle the most appropriate response.)

    (0) Not at all important
    (1) Somewhat important
    (2) Neither important nor unimportant
    (3) Somewhat important
    (4) Very important

21. Circle the number that corresponds to the statement that best describes your sexual experience.

    (1) Entirely heterosexual
    (2) Largely heterosexual, but some homosexual experience
    (3) Largely heterosexual, but considerable homosexual experience
    (4) Equally heterosexual and homosexual
    (5) Largely homosexual, but considerable heterosexual experience
    (6) Largely homosexual, but some heterosexual experience
    (7) Entirely homosexual

22. Circle the number that corresponds to the statement that best describes your sexual desires.

    (1) Entirely heterosexual
    (2) Largely heterosexual, but some homosexual desire
    (3) Largely heterosexual, but considerable homosexual desire
    (4) Equally heterosexual and homosexual desires
    (5) Largely homosexual, but considerable heterosexual desire
    (6) Largely homosexual, but some heterosexual desire
    (7) Entirely homosexual

Note. From Taylor, Rosen, and Leiblum (1994). Copyright 1994 by Plenum Publishing Corp. Reprinted by permission.

TABLE 6.3. Sexual Desire Inventory

This questionnaire asks about your level of sexual desire. By desire, we mean interest in or wish for sexual activity. For each item, please circle the number that best shows your thoughts and feelings. Your answers will be private.

1. Over the last month, *how often* would you have liked to engage in sexual activity with a partner? (Sexual activities with a partner may include such things as touching each others genitals, giving or receiving oral stimulation, intercourse, etc.)

   (0) Not at all   (4) Twice a week
   (1) Once a month   (5) 3 to 4 times a week
   (2) Once every 2 weeks   (6) Once a day
   (3) Once a week   (7) More than once a day

2. Over the last month, *how often* have you had sexual thoughts involving a partner?

   (0) Not at all   (4) 3 to 4 times a week
   (1) Once or twice a month   (5) Once a day
   (2) Once a week   (6) A couple of times a day
   (3) Twice a week   (7) Many times a day

3. When you have sexual thoughts, *how strong* is your desire to engage in sexual behavior with a partner?

0	1	2	3	4	5	6	7	8
no desire								strong desire

4. When you first see an attractive person, *how strong* is your sexual desire?

0	1	2	3	4	5	6	7	8
no desire								strong desire

5. When you spend time with an attractive person (e.g., at work or school), *how strong* is your sexual desire?

0	1	2	3	4	5	6	7	8
no desire								strong desire

6. When you are in romantic situations (such as a candlelit dinner, a walk on the beach, etc.), *how strong* is your sexual desire?

0	1	2	3	4	5	6	7	8
no desire								strong desire

(continued)

TABLE 6.3. (*continued*)

7. *How strong* is your desire to engage in sexual activity with a partner?

0	1	2	3	4	5	6	7	8
no desire								strong desire

8. *How important* is it for you to fulfill your sexual desire through activity with a partner?

0	1	2	3	4	5	6	7	8
not important								extremely important

9. Compared to other people of your age and sex, how would you rate your desire to behave sexually with a partner?

0	1	2	3	4	5	6	7	8
much less desire								much more desire

10. Over the last month, *how often* would you *have liked* to behave sexually by yourself (e.g., masturbating, touching your genitals, etc.)?

(0) Not at all
(1) Once a month
(2) Once every 2 weeks
(3) Once a week

(4) Twice a week
(5) 3 to 4 times a week
(6) Once a day
(7) More than once a day

11. *How strong* is your desire to engage in sexual activity by yourself?

0	1	2	3	4	5	6	7	8
no desire								strong desire

12. *How important* is it for you to fulfill your sexual desire through self-stimulation activities?

0	1	2	3	4	5	6	7	8
no desire								strong desire

13. Compared to other people of your age and sex, how would you rate your desire to behave sexually by yourself?

0	1	2	3	4	5	6	7	8
much less desire								much more desire

TABLE 6.3. *(continued)*

14. *How long* could you go comfortably without having sexual activity of some kind?

(0) Forever	(5) A week
(1) A year or two	(6) A few days
(2) Several months	(7) One day
(3) A month	(8) Less than one day
(4) A few weeks	

Note. From Spector, Carey, and Steinberg (1996). Copyright 1996 by Brunner/Mazel. Reprinted by permission.

should score higher on the solitary desire dimension. The SDI should also be helpful in the evaluation of change over time.

INTERNATIONAL INDEX OF ERECTILE FUNCTION (IIEF)

The IIEF (Rosen et al., 1997) is a 15-item self-report measure of erectile functioning that is psychometrically sound, sensitive to treatment changes, and available in 10 languages: Danish, Dutch, English (American, Australian, British), Finnish, French, German, Italian, Norwegian, Spanish, and Swedish. (Validation of the scale in Arabic, Chinese, and Portuguese, among others, is underway!) The IIEF has separate items for achieving and maintaining erections, and it assesses the ability to achieve erections in nonintercourse sexual activity. There is one item that asks about the respondent's confidence in being able to achieve and maintain an erection, a psychological dimension shown to be related to treatment outcome (Rosen, Leiblum, & Spector, 1994). The IIEF assesses current sexual functioning in five domains: erectile functioning, orgasmic functioning, sexual desire, intercourse satisfaction, and overall satisfaction. The internal consistency for each of the five domains measured by the IIEF has been established, and test–retest stability is also strong. All five domains, except the sexual desire domain, can discriminate between men with and without erectile problems. (As noted earlier, we prefer the SDI for direct assessment of desire difficulties in men as well as women.) Based on outcome studies examining treatment of erectile disorder by sildenafil citrate, the sensitivity and specificity to treatment changes were demonstrated. Advantages of the IIEF are that it takes less than 15 minutes to complete, and it is comprehensive and easily scored. Assessment of other components associated with sexual function and of the relationship by the IIEF is limited. Another limitation of the IIEF is that it has only been validated with heterosexual patients, and that the standard instructions define sexual intercourse as "penile–vaginal penetration," making it less applicable to gay and bisexual men.

INVENTORY OF DYADIC HETEROSEXUAL PREFERENCES (IDHP; SEE TABLE 6.4)

The IDHP (Purnine, Carey, & Jorgensen, 1996) is a reliable and valid measure of individuals' sexual behavior preferences. Factor analysis has confirmed that its 27 items reflect six distinct areas of behavior preference: erotophilia, use of contraceptives, conventionality, use of erotica, use of drugs/alcohol, and romantic foreplay. It is less useful as a measure of treatment outcome but very useful as a measure of interpersonal processes in a couple. The instructions ask individuals how they would like things to be in their current relationship. Subjects not currently involved in an intimate relationship can respond according to how they would like things to be in a hypothetical relationship.

We have used the IDHP to explore compatibility and communication between partners (Purnine & Carey, 1999). We do this by having partners complete the IDHP twice: once identifying their own preferences, and a second time identifying what they think are their partner's preferences. This is an intriguing exercise and yields information about the extent to which preferences are shared, and the extent to which partners understand one another. We have found in our research that sexual satisfaction in both male and female partners was associated with men understanding their partner's preferences (Purnine & Carey, 1997). The influential role of a male understanding his partner's preferences was strong and accounted for 51% and 63%, respectively, of variance in men's and women's sexual satisfaction! Agreement, it turns out, is less important than understanding.

Not surprisingly, other research with the IDHP reveals that preferences vary as a function of age and gender (Purnine & Carey, 1998). For example, women's preference for romantic foreplay is stronger than men's, and men's preference for using erotica and combining alcohol and drug use with sex is stronger than women's. A somewhat counterintuitive finding of our research was that older couples tend to be less conventional than their younger couples, for example, they are more inclined toward the use of erotica.

Although this scale was developed for use with heterosexual partners, it may also be useful with gay, lesbian, or bisexual partners.

DYADIC ADJUSTMENT SCALE (DAS)

The DAS (Spanier, 1976) is particularly valuable for assessing problem areas within a couple's interaction outside of the sexual domain. The DAS consists of a list of 32 items designed to assess the quality of the relationship as perceived by married or cohabiting couples. Partners complete the questionnaire separately. Scoring yields four subscales and a total score; however, we tend to use only the total score in our work. It provides a general measure of marital/cohabiting satisfaction. According to Jensen et al. (1987), the instructions of

TABLE 6.4. Index of Dyadic Heterosexual Preferences (IDHP)

Instructions: Please read the following statements carefully and indicate how much you agree or disagree that the statement is true for you. Respond to each item as you would actually like things to be in relations with your partner. Feel free to ask about any statement that is not clear to you. Please respond to all items. THERE ARE NO RIGHT OR WRONG ANSWERS. *RESPOND AS TRUTHFULLY AS POSSIBLE.*

1. I would like to initiate sex.

strongly agree	agree	somewhat agree	somewhat disagree	disagree	strongly disagree
6	5	4	3	2	1

2. An intimate, romantic dinner together would be a real turn on to me.

strongly agree	agree	somewhat agree	somewhat disagree	disagree	strongly disagree
6	5	4	3	2	1

3. Using spermicide would spoil sex for me.

strongly agree	agree	somewhat agree	somewhat disagree	disagree	strongly disagree
6	5	4	3	2	1

4. I would like to use a vibrator or other sexual toy (or aid) during sex.

strongly agree	agree	somewhat agree	somewhat disagree	disagree	strongly disagree
6	5	4	3	2	1

5. I would prefer to have sex under the bedcovers and with the lights on.

strongly agree	agree	somewhat agree	somewhat disagree	disagree	strongly disagree
6	5	4	3	2	1

6. Having myself or my partner use a condom would not spoil sex for me.

strongly agree	agree	somewhat agree	somewhat disagree	disagree	strongly disagree
6	5	4	3	2	1

7. Having sex in rooms other than the bedroom would turn me on.

strongly agree	agree	somewhat agree	somewhat disagree	disagree	strongly disagree
6	5	4	3	2	1

(continued)

TABLE 6.4. (*continued*)

8.   I would prefer to have sex everyday.

strongly agree	agree	somewhat agree	somewhat disagree	disagree	strongly disagree
6	5	4	3	2	1

9.   Looking at sexually explicit books and movies would turn me on.

strongly agree	agree	somewhat agree	somewhat disagree	disagree	strongly disagree
6	5	4	3	2	1

10.   I would not enjoy looking at my partner's genitals.

strongly agree	agree	somewhat agree	somewhat disagree	disagree	strongly disagree
6	5	4	3	2	1

11.   I would like to have sex after a day at the beach.

strongly agree	agree	somewhat agree	somewhat disagree	disagree	strongly disagree
6	5	4	3	2	1

12.   I would like to mix alcohol and sex.

strongly agree	agree	somewhat agree	somewhat disagree	disagree	strongly disagree
6	5	4	3	2	1

13.   Using a contraceptive would not affect my sexual satisfaction or pleasure.

strongly agree	agree	somewhat agree	somewhat disagree	disagree	strongly disagree
6	5	4	3	2	1

14.   I would enjoy having sex after smoking marijuana.

strongly agree	agree	somewhat agree	somewhat disagree	disagree	strongly disagree
6	5	4	3	2	1

15.   I would prefer to have sex while using drugs that make me feel aroused.

strongly agree	agree	somewhat agree	somewhat disagree	disagree	strongly disagree
6	5	4	3	2	1

16.   I would enjoy having sex outdoors.

strongly agree	agree	somewhat agree	somewhat disagree	disagree	strongly disagree
6	5	4	3	2	1

TABLE 6.4. *(continued)*

17. My preferred time for having sex is in the morning.

strongly agree	agree	somewhat agree	somewhat disagree	disagree	strongly disagree
6	5	4	3	2	1

18. Swimming in the nude with my partner would be a turn-on.

strongly agree	agree	somewhat agree	somewhat disagree	disagree	strongly disagree
6	5	4	3	2	1

19. I would enjoy dressing in sexy/revealing clothes to arouse my partner.

strongly agree	agree	somewhat agree	somewhat disagree	disagree	strongly disagree
6	5	4	3	2	1

20. I would like to mix drugs and sex.

strongly agree	agree	somewhat agree	somewhat disagree	disagree	strongly disagree
6	5	4	3	2	1

21. I would get turned on if my partner touched my chest and nipples.

strongly agree	agree	somewhat agree	somewhat disagree	disagree	strongly disagree
6	5	4	3	2	1

22. I would prefer to avoid having sex during my (partner's) period.

strongly agree	agree	somewhat agree	somewhat disagree	disagree	strongly disagree
6	5	4	3	2	1

23. I would not enjoy having my partner look at my genitals.

strongly agree	agree	somewhat agree	somewhat disagree	disagree	strongly disagree
6	5	4	3	2	1

24. Sexually explicit books and movies are disgusting to me.

strongly agree	agree	somewhat agree	somewhat disagree	disagree	strongly disagree
6	5	4	3	2	1

25. I would find deep kissing with the tongue quite arousing.

strongly agree	agree	somewhat agree	somewhat disagree	disagree	strongly disagree
6	5	4	3	2	1

(continued)

TABLE 6.4. (continued)

26. Using a vaginal lubricant (K-Y jelly) would spoil sex for me.

strongly agree	agree	somewhat agree	somewhat disagree	disagree	strongly disagree
6	5	4	3	2	1

27. Watching erotic movies with my partner would turn me on.

strongly agree	agree	somewhat agree	somewhat disagree	disagree	strongly disagree
6	5	4	3	2	1

Note. From Purnine, Carey, and Jorgensen (1996). Copyright 1996 by Elsevier Science Ltd. Reprinted by permission.

the DAS are at a seventh-grade reading level, whereas the items themselves are at the eighth-grade reading level; thus, it should be possible to use the DAS with most patients. Research suggests that the DAS is valid and reliable (see Spanier, 1976). Most people can complete the DAS in 15 minutes, and it can be scored in about 5 minutes. The DAS has proven to be consistently valuable over time. In fact, in a study of frequently cited sources in human sexology (Thompson, Lake, & Richards, 1994) the original paper on the DAS was listed as the most frequently cited article.

Specialized Measures

Some measures are useful for special circumstances. For example, patients who have had multiple partners or engage in other risky sexual practices may require more detailed assessment of HIV-related knowledge risk. Persons who present with other psychological and psychosexual concerns might profit from an omnibus assessment. Therefore, we describe several measures that may be useful to have available.

The *HIV-Knowledge Questionnaire* (HIV-K-Q; Carey, Morrison-Beedy, & Johnson, 1997) was developed to measure knowledge about the transmission, prevention, and consequences of HIV infection. This measure has been demonstrated to be reliable and valid; understandable to those with an eighth-grade education or less; and appropriate for use regardless of respondent age, gender, race/ethnicity, and sexual orientation. The measure takes less than 5 minutes to complete and can be helpful for the assessment and evaluation of focused HIV-education efforts and as a conversation starter about HIV and other STDs.

The *Sexual Opinion Survey* (SOS; Fisher, 1988; Fisher, Byrne, White, & Kelley, 1988) is also used to aid our understanding of the individual. The SOS consists of 21 items intended to assess affective and evaluative responses to a range of sexual stimuli (autosexual, heterosexual, and homosexual behavior; sexual fantasy; visual sexual stimuli) (Fisher, 1988). Each of these 21 items describes a sexual situation and a negative or positive affective response; patients then indicate the extent to which they agree (or disagree) with the affective response. Research suggests that the SOS is valid and reliable, and norms are available (Fisher et al., 1988). Most people can complete the SOS in 10 minutes or less, and it can be scored in about half that time.

The *Derogatis Sexual Functioning Inventory* (DSFI; Derogatis & Melisaratos, 1979) is an omnibus scale (245 items) of sexual functioning but it remains a valuable assessment tool despite its age and length. We find it useful when we are not quite sure of all the possible dimensions of an individual's sexual problem, for example, cases where there may be sexual dysfunction but also possible paraphilia or very unusual or rigid views of sexuality. The DSFI measures 10 domains considered to be essential to effective sexual functioning: information, experience, drive, attitudes, psychological symptoms, affect, gender-role definition, fantasy, body image, and sexual satisfaction. One of the subscales, the Psychological Symptoms subtest, is a distinct psychological instrument also known as the Brief Symptom Inventory (BSI; Derogatis & Spencer, 1982). Scores on the BSI yield nine subscales (Somatization, Obsessive–Compulsive, Interpersonal Sensitivity, Depression, Anxiety, Hostility, Phobic Anxiety, Paranoid Ideation, and Psychoticism), as well as three global indices (Global Severity Index, Positive Symptom Distress Index, and Positive Symptom Total). The BSI may come in handy with patients for whom you suspect some interfering psychopathology. Research suggests that the DSFI is reliable and valid, and norms are available (see Derogatis, 1975). The DSFI does require high school reading skills and takes 45 minutes to complete; scoring is complicated. Therefore, we do not recommend this as a routine measure, but it can be helpful in some situations.

Concluding Comments on the Use of Self-Report Questionnaires

Although we encourage you to use carefully selected self-report questionnaires in your work, we also wish to be clear about their limitations. Such measures should never be used blindly or without a careful interview. Moreover, we wish to be clear about "traditional" psychological measures such as the MMPI (Hathaway & McKinley, 1967) or the Rorschach inkblot test (Exner, 1986). These measures have *not* been found useful for diagnosing the presence of sexual dysfunction or for delineating its etiology (Conte, 1986). Therefore, we discourage their use, unless it is for some other purpose for which that instrument has been demonstrated to be reliable and valid.

Psychophysiological Assessment

Psychophysiology permits inferences about psychological processes that are based upon physiological measures (Cacioppo & Tassinary, 1990). Thus, if available, these measures can be powerful tools in your assessment armamentarium. Among other strengths, psychophysiological measures tend to be less susceptible to the distortions and biases that can occur with interviews and questionnaires. In addition, psychophysiological measures permit a better understanding of the physiological underpinnings, and sometimes the actual mechanisms, of a dysfunction.

We use the term "psychophysiological" in the narrow sense of noninvasive, surface measures. Certainly, one can construe the assessment of hormonal levels in the blood as a psychophysiological measure. However, we refer to measures that are invasive and/or that require medical expertise and supervision as "medical measures" (discussed later).

In practice, psychophysiological methods are used infrequently because, first, these methods require significant technical skill to achieve a minimal level of competence. Only a limited number of training programs provide the opportunities for clinicians to acquire such skills. Second, the psychophysiological recording apparatus and supplies are expensive, at least initially; in a general clinical practice, it is often not feasible to add this expense (which almost certainly would not be reimbursable) to an assessment protocol. Finally, the procedures remain largely "experimental" in the sense that they have not been used extensively in clinical practice, especially in the use of female physiological evaluations.

Nevertheless, practitioners who have the opportunity to acquire the necessary skills and envision a practice large enough to support the investment will need to know more about the psychophysiological options. All practitioners will benefit from a better understanding of these approaches to communicate with patients and physicians, and to know when such studies can be helpful. To our knowledge, psychophysiological studies are rarely done with women for clinical purposes (research, however, is increasing). Studies with men have continued to use the penile strain gauge technology with nocturnal penile tumescence (NPT), daytime arousal, and nap studies.

Nocturnal Penile Tumescence Studies

The physiological recording of NPT, usually in a full sleep laboratory or center, is still considered the "gold standard" of differential diagnosis in men. Briefly, the rationale for this procedure is as follows: If a man can obtain an erection during sleep (which most men do on four or five occasions per night) but cannot obtain an erection during partner stimulation, it is assumed that the source of the erectile dysfunction is "psychogenic" (or "functional"). In contrast, if a man cannot obtain an erection at night, it has been assumed that his dysfunction is "organic."

Despite the promise of NPT, there are still several important challenges to its use and interpretation. An extended discussion of these challenges is provided elsewhere (see Meisler & Carey, 1990), and we wish to mention only two here. First, from a purely technical viewpoint, data indicate that NPT may be influenced by sleep problems (e.g., apnea, hypopnea, or periodic leg movements) not routinely assessed in the typical NPT evaluation. These sleep parameters may produce artifacts that can interfere with interpretation of NPT tracings. Second, from a practical perspective, NPT monitoring can be very costly. The procedure may require expensive equipment and necessitate that a patient spend two or three nights in a sleep center. As a result, this assessment procedure has been well beyond the financial means of most patients.

One pragmatic alternative to the sleep laboratory has been the use of the RigiScan. The RigiScan is usually available in urology clinics that specialize in the treatment of male sexual problems. This device is used at home and is about the size of a videotape. It is worn by the patient in a thigh holster with two lead wires ending in circular transducers attached to the penis. The RigiScan records a full night's penis circumference and rigidity changes. The record is then downloaded into a computer and displays number of erections, and fullness and rigidity of each erection.

Another intriguing alternative to full-night NPT assessment is assessing erectile functioning during morning naps! Webb, Agnew, and Sternthal (1966) reported that the electroencephalographic (EEG) patterns of subjects who napped in the early morning resemble sleep stages from the second half of the night, with prominent REM sleep. This finding is important because REM sleep has been strongly associated with sleep erections (Rosen & Beck, 1988). Moses, Hord, Lubin, Johnson, and Naitoh (1975) also found that subjects who took brief naps following sleep deprivation resumed their previously interrupted REM cycles at the next sleep onset, with REM onset frequently occurring within 10 minutes of nap onset.

We set out to explore the value of penile tumescence monitoring during daytime naps. In our first study (Gordon & Carey, 1993), 7 young men took a 3-hour morning nap, while sleep and penile tumescence measures were recorded. All subjects slept well and experienced at least one sleep erection with significant circumference change ($M = 37.3$ mm). In a second study, (Gordon & Carey, 1995), we included 30 men whose ages were more representative of patients in sexual health clinics. The men reduced their normal sleep time to increase the likelihood that they would experience REM sleep. They then reported to an outpatient setting for an early morning nap, during which sleep and penile tumescence measures were recorded. All men were able to sleep during at least one of their two recording sessions, 80% experienced REM sleep, and 73% experienced tumescence episodes. The magnitude of the erections would reduce concerns about the presence of organic pathology and obviate the need for a more expensive NPT study. Although these results suggest that monitoring tumescence during naps is useful as an inexpensive screening approach, this approach has not yet been widely adopted. We review this research here because it may prove practical in some settings where assessment of male functioning is done frequently.

Daytime Arousal Studies

Measuring sexual arousal directly (i.e., in response to erotic stimulation) can be extremely valuable; indeed, it is the lack of such a response that is often reported as the problem in erectile dysfunction. Psychophysiological measurement of sexual arousal offers an objective view of a person's response to erotic stimuli. Psychophysiological studies (Libman et al., 1989; Sakheim, Barlow, Abrahamson, & Beck, 1987; Wincze et al., 1988) have provided valuable information for the assessment process. This is an especially valuable approach for assessing men who neither masturbate nor use erotica on a regular basis. For example, Wincze et al. (1988) found that exposing some dysfunctional men to erotic stimulation resulted in full erection responses, even though those men reported an inability to obtain an erection. Such data can be critically helpful in formulating a case.

In brief, our procedure uses videotapes of erotic stimulation presented for approximately 8 to 10 minutes. The viewing time is longer than is often noted in research studies, but in our clinical settings, it allows a person to relax and get mentally involved in the stimulus presentation.

Throughout the procedure, the patient is seated in a separate room in privacy. Stimuli are selected carefully, after the interview, so that they are appropriate to a person's sexual orientation and exclude material a patient might find offensive. Using a mercury strain gauge, we can measure precisely the amount of tumescence and the point in the videotape at which the tumescence appears. The debriefing following this assessment procedure can be especially valuable; we use it to help us to understand the patient's cognitive reaction to erotic stimulation. We ask questions about the patient's ability to concentrate on the erotic stimuli and his emotional reaction to the stimuli. For example, one 56-year-old patient experiencing erectile difficulties expressed detachment from the erotic stimulation: "That stuff doesn't bother me. I know they are just acting, and I need the real thing." Further inquiry revealed that this patient had very limited use of erotic fantasy and, in fact, felt it was "wrong" to fantasize. The conflict between his "obligation" to have sex with his wife and his restricted views about sexual expressions later became the focus of therapy.

When you see your first patient, it is unlikely that you will have the technical expertise or laboratory equipment needed to conduct a thorough psychophysiological assessment. However, if you anticipate that you will be conducting a large number of assessments, we would encourage you to obtain this equipment and to seek further, supervised training.

Medical Evaluation

In addition to the information you obtain from the interview, self-report questionnaires, and psychophysiological evaluation, you will also need to know (1) when (and how) to refer a patient for medical testing and (2) how to interpret and integrate into you case formulation the results of the most common medical tests.

As mentioned earlier, information about a patient's medical history and visits to physicians should be a routine part of your initial screening interview. As we have also discussed previously, your interview may be supplemented with a medical history questionnaire that asks for basic information about chronic and acute medical conditions, medication use, surgical history, congenital disorders, hospitalizations, significant medical problems within the extended family, and visits to physicians. This will save you time during your interview and help to alert you to important medical considerations.

Even when you have conducted a careful interview and collected additional information with self-report questionnaires, it may be necessary to refer your patient for further medical evaluation. Indeed, we believe that it is good practice to refer any patient for a medical workup if he or she has not recently been examined. Clients who describe pain, discomfort, bleeding, discharge, or any other unusual symptoms that have not been recently evaluated should be referred to a physician before proceeding with a psychosocially oriented treatment approach. In our view, it is best to be conservative and to refer patients to a physician if there is any concern whatsoever.

When a patient has had a recent medical evaluation and the dysfunction is manifested only under certain circumstances, or with certain partners, then it is less likely that further medical evaluation is necessary. However, you should continue to be vigilant for complications that may require additional medical consultation.

How to Identify a Medical Consultant

It is extremely important to select your medical consultants with great care. We suggest your selection should be based upon the following considerations:

1. Select a physician who is willing to work cooperatively with you and to respect your contributions. We discourage you from working with a physician who takes over the case and begins treatment without consulting you. For

example, if you refer a patient for evaluation of male erectile disorder, you should expect that the consultant will get back to you before initiating treatment.

2. Try to find a physician who is willing, within reasonable limits, to educate you regarding his or her specialty. Professionals differ with regard to their ability to communicate knowledge.

3. Try to assess the consultant's interpersonal skills or, as they are traditionally referred to, his or her "bedside manner." It would reflect negatively on your judgment if you referred your patients to a physician who is aloof, cold, or even disrespectful. We have heard reports regarding all types of unprofessional behavior. For example, one report was of a physician grabbing an overweight male patient in the abdomen and stating, "You are too fat to have sex, so why bother?" We have also known of physicians who have encouraged patients to have extramarital affairs to solve sexual problems.

4. Try to determine the physician's competence and comfort with sexual problems. Medicine is a large and complex field; being trained as a physician, even as a genital specialist (i.e., in gynecology or urology), does not guarantee current knowledge or comfort with sexual problems. It is important to discuss with potential consultants their self-efficacy and comfort in dealing with sexual complaints. If possible, it is worthwhile to check with other experienced sex therapists regarding good consultants.

When you deem it important to obtain additional medical evaluation, you will need to coordinate this referral. We suggest a two-stage approach. First, we have found it helpful to call the physician. If you are calling a physician for the first time, you may want to tell the receptionist that you have a patient referral; ask whether you can have the "back number," as most physicians have a separate line for such calls. If you do not go to this extra trouble, you may have to wait several days for a return call, since most physicians are busy. Once you have established telephone contact and determined that the physician is an appropriate referral, you will want to provide him or her with a *brief* written report to guide the assessment.

It is important that your written referral be brief and outline the specific reason for your referral. Again, avoid psychojargon! An example of a letter referring one of your patients is shown in Figure 6.1.

Interpreting Medical Test Results

After you have referred a patient for a medical consultation, you will need to integrate the results of this evaluation into your assessment. To do this, you need to be able to interpret test results. A nonphysician should, of course, rely on a physician's interpretation of medical test results. However, we believe that there are at least three reasons why you should learn the basics about the

RE: David Longwood, D.O.B.: 3/1/33

Dear Dr. Quigley:

I am referring Mr. David Longwood to you for evaluation of possible medical factors that may be contributing to his problem of erectile dysfunction. Mr. Longwood has experienced intermittent erectile dysfunction for the past five years but this has been a consistent problem for the past year.

Mr. Longwood is a very bright, professional man and is in a very satisfying long-term marriage. I believe that his sexual problem could have been precipitated by job-related stress but I would also like to rule out any possible medical factors. I would greatly appreciate it if you would examine Mr. Longwood and inform me of any medical factors that may be affecting his sexual functioning.

Sincerely,

Dr. Conroy

FIGURE 6.1. An example of a referral letter.

most common procedures, tests, and results. First, this knowledge will help you to obtain the most crucial information in an efficient manner when you communicate with your consultants. Second, this knowledge will allow you to prepare patients for the tests they are likely to undergo, and to discuss the results of these tests as they affect your formulation and treatment planning. Third, such knowledge will enhance your understanding of your patient, which will help you to be a better therapist.

ENDOCRINE MEASURES

Hormonal levels may be important to the sexual health of both men and women. In interpreting the results of hormonal levels, several factors are important. First, it is important to remember that levels may vary depending on the assay procedure used; thus, levels typically vary somewhat across laboratories. Second, values should be understood as falling along a continuum of possible values, and the concept of a normal *range* is important. Third, it is critical to know the measurement units that are being used.

In women, estradiol is considered important. Typically, results are presented in picograms per milliliter (pg/ml). Because estradiol values fluctuate with the phases of the menstrual cycle, menstrual phase should be known when the sample is obtained and interpreted. The normal range of plasma estradiol during the first 10 days of the cycle averages 50 pg/ml; during the last 20 days, it averages 125 pg/ml. (Men normally average 20 pg/ml at all times.) Values below the normal range for a particular phase may adversely affect vaginal lubrication.

In men, testosterone and prolactin are important. For testosterone, values are typically expressed in nanograms per deciliter (ng/dl) or in nanograms per milliliter (ng/ml). In laboratories with which we work, the normal range in men is usually from 280 to 1,100 ng/dl, or from 2.8 to 11.0 ng/ml. (The normal range in women is 6.0–86.0 ng/dl.) Testosterone values need to be obtained during the early morning, because testosterone in males responds to a diurnal cycle, with the highest values recorded during the morning. You should also know that testosterone values are usually expressed as total testosterone; this includes both bioavailable and inactive testosterone. The bioavailable testosterone that influences sexual behavior is a fraction of the total and is composed of both free testosterone and albumin-bound testosterone.

Prolactin is a pituitary hormone that causes the breasts to enlarge and to secrete milk; it is also believed to be important for evaluating sexual desire in men. Specifically, higher levels of prolactin have been associated with decreased sexual desire. The normal range for prolactin in men and women (except for women during pregnancy and while nursing, when higher levels are observed) is 0–20 ng/ml. A value greater than 20 ng/ml warrants a repeat test, because it may intimate, among other conditions, the presence of a pituitary tumor.

As we have worked with physicians, we have found that there are several reference books that help to understand test values, medications, and diseases. Beers and Berkow's (1999) *The Merck Manual of Diagnosis and Therapy* is an excellent reference book that is intended for physicians but can be helpful for nonphysicians as well; it is available in most medical school bookstores and is revised often. Another handbook that we have found helpful is Levine's (1996) *Pocket Guide to Commonly Prescribed Drugs*, because many of our older patients often take numerous medication. Given the rapidly changing science of medicine, you will need to restock your library every few years to remain current.

Conjoint Interview and Case Formulation: Session 3

The third interview normally includes both partners. (An exception to this may occur if one individual's needs are so overwhelming that individual therapy is indicated prior to couple therapy, as in the earlier case example). The interview with both partners should begin in an open-ended manner to determine what changes and conversations may have occurred since the last session. A couple's response to this approach is important diagnostically because it provides an understanding of how the couple approaches and discusses important problematic topics. You can observe which partner takes responsibility for what, and how effectively each person communicates his or her needs.

Consider, also, that a couple may be overwhelmed with recently occurring problems or stressors, such as job loss or death in the family. Obviously, it is important to acknowledge nonsexual issues that may preoccupy patients and distract them from the current focus of the assessment. The remainder of the third session should be spent providing your formulation, identifying treatment goals (sexual and nonsexual), outlining therapy plans, and explaining details regarding the initial stages of therapy. To further facilitate rapport, maximize therapy compliance, and avoid backsliding, you should ask each partner how he or she feels about the plan and what problems each anticipates as barriers to progress.

Elements of the third assessment session might be as follows:

Assumptions

As before, it is useful to begin with assumptions in the most helpful direction. For example, you may find it helpful to assume the following:

- Couple has not discussed previous interviews.
- Couple has trouble discussing sexual matters and is embarrassed.
- There may still be a crisis.
- Correct terminology is still not well understood.
- Sexual attitudes are rigid and conservative.
- Avoidance of sex will occur because of fear and discomfort.

These assumptions position the therapist to approach the third assessment session with caution to counteract a possible therapist-pleasing presentation on the part of the couple. Thus, although a couple may present as though "things seem better," the crisis most likely still exists and needs attention. Certainly, the therapist should not approach the couple pessimistically but should realistically approach all issues.

Goals

You should also establish goals for this session; possible goals include the following:

- Review your own observations and formulations.
- Invite the couple to identify inconsistencies between your observations and formulation and theirs.
- Outline and begin a therapy plan.
- Obtain the couple's commitment to follow the therapy plan by discussing potential compliance problems ahead of time.
- Encourage the couple to begin conceptualizing problem as learned and "situational," and discourage partners from blaming one another.

Process

Process issues continue to be important. Thus you may want to cover the following points:

- Ask the couple whether there are any developments since your last meeting.
- Ask the couple what they have discussed: Why or why not?
- Ask whether there are any doubts or issues to be discussed before therapy begins.
- Ask the couple whether there are any anticipated difficulties in participating in therapy with you as therapist. (Are there concerns regarding the therapist's gender, age, or race?)

Interview Structure and Content

The third session may be ordered as follows:

1. After consideration of process issues, begin the interview by defining the problem, indicating possible contributing factors, and acknowledging that you will continue to collect information as therapy starts. Ask each partner to comment on and clarify any misunderstandings or disagreements.

2. Ask each partner to discuss his or her reaction to a sexual encounter when it is thought to be a failure.

3. Outline the therapy plan; if possible, try to discuss all stages of therapy. Emphasize, in detail, what the first stage will involve—this will establish hope. Be sure to ask the couple to identify any anticipated problems and to commit to the initial step (i.e., set a specific date and time for your next meeting).

For many patients, further assessment information will be needed, such as psychological testing, psychophysiological assessment, and/or medical evaluation. If this is the case, then therapy instructions may have to be postponed until the assessment picture is completed. (Later in this chapter, we discuss the integration of interview data with information obtained from other methods.) It is very important to explain the nature of and need for further assessment, so that a patient does not get discouraged or frustrated.

The interview is the most common procedure for assessing sexual problems. Over the years, as our clinical sophistication and knowledge base have increased, the interview procedure for assessment of sexual problems has become more structured and standardized. Thus, today's interviewing methods yield more valuable information then ever before; we are more knowledgeable about the complexities of sexual functioning. The remainder of this chapter focuses on integrating multiple sources of information and recognizing special challenges to the assessment process.

Integrating Multiple Data Sources into a Coherent Case Formulation

We mentioned at the beginning of this chapter that one of the goals of the assessment is to develop a coherent case formulation (i.e., a working hypothesis of the etiology of the problem). This formulation should relate all aspects of a patient's complaints to one another and explain why the individual has developed these difficulties (Carey et al., 1984). One purpose of this formulation is to aid you in the development of a treatment plan. A second purpose is to communicate to your patients that (1) their problem is an understandable one given their physiology, medical history, life experiences, and so forth (i.e., they are not crazy or perverted); (2) there is reason for hope and optimism; and (3) you have a conceptual "road map" and rationale upon which to build a therapeutic plan. Finally, developing a case formulation allows you to check with the patient to see whether you have obtained all necessary information, and whether the information that you have is correct.

One of the more challenging aspects of sex therapy is integrating multiple levels of influence (i.e., biological, psychological, dyadic, cultural) into a coherent case formulation. Despite its difficulty, a biopsychosocial case formulation captures the richness of sexual function and dysfunction. Patients are more likely to agree to try a psychosocial approach if you recognize that biological causes are not irrelevant, but point out that they may be compensated for or overridden. A patient also more likely to agree to try a psychosocial approach if you inquire about and recognize specific dyadic and sociocultural influences. You need to be sensitive to specific rituals and habits that a couple has established, as well as to ethnic, cultural, or religious traditions.

Your case formulation should include biological, psychological, and social areas even if you believe that one area does not contribute to the problem at the moment. It is difficult to predict the future, and you will have laid the groundwork should additional information become available and/or future developments occur. Moreover, this comprehensive approach to case formulation will give the patient confidence that you have considered all possibilities. Indirectly, you communicate to the patient that he or she should also think about the problem in a multifaceted, biopsychosocial framework.

To illustrate how you might present your information to a couple, we provide the following script based upon a composite of cases.

"Mr. and Mrs. Anthony, I want to use this session to review all of the information I have gathered and outline for you a possible treatment plan. The problem that you are concerned about is Mr. Anthony's difficulty with being unable to ejaculate. This, of course, is very troubling because you both expressed a strong desire to have children.

"I want to point out some very positive findings in your situation. You both have expressed a very strong attraction and desire for each other and there do not appear to be any serious marital conflicts. Furthermore, the results of your medical examination, Mr. Anthony, are completely normal. There do not appear to be any medical factors complicating the picture. I believe that Dr. Jones reassured you that the medication you are taking for your skin problem is not causing the problem associated with ejaculation.

"In my assessment of both of you, I have covered a lot of possible factors that can cause sexual problems. Most of these areas we have talked about did not seem to apply to your situation. What did seem important, however, were two factors:

"First, both of you work a great many hours during the week and, because Mr. Anthony has a long commute, he does not get home until very late. You both agree that sex during the week is almost impossible because there is little time together. Your weekends seem to be equally busy and both of you feel you need more relaxed, fun time together.

"Second, another possible factor is Mr. Anthony's difficulty in leaving his work even when he is home. Mr. Anthony, you reported that your mind is always problem solving and thinking of many issues. In fact, you said it is difficult for you to relax even when you do go on vacation. When it comes to sex, you said you are always worrying about ejaculation and rarely just enjoy the experience. This style of thinking is most likely interfering with sex and is something we should work on in therapy.

"So, overall, I am suggesting that there are three factors that, together, appear to be causing and maintaining the ejaculation difficulty. The first factor involves the lack of time combined with exhaustion resulting from working such long hours; this factor leaves you little time to develop conditions conducive to a relaxing and fulfilling sex life. The second factor involves preoccupation with work matters, even during sex. And the third factor, what I will call performance pressure, results from the first two factors."

[At this point, the therapist should pause and ask how each person feels about the formulation and ask if either partner feels anything has been left out or not considered. Following any discussion of the formulation, the therapist then outlines the specific strategies for addressing each identified treatment issue.]

"If you agree that these factors do appear to be responsible, at least in part, for the ejaculation concerns, here's how I'd suggest we proceed. First, I think we need to work together to protect time to invest in your relationship, when both of you feel that you can truly relax and be there for each other. We will need to review other commitments and be creative in time management. I have some brief readings on the matter of time management that I'd like each of you to read in advance of our discussion.

"Second, I'd like to work individually with you, Mr. Anthony, to help you to manage your thinking about work in a way that works better for you. We will do some stress management work around physical relaxation and elimination of unwanted thoughts. I will ask you to practice a stress management approach that is comfortable for you, such as relaxation exercises, yoga, or meditation, depending on your preferences. I think you will enjoy this, and see benefits in other aspects of you life as well.

"When we have completed the time and stress management efforts, which should not take too long, we can focus on specific sexual exercises that I will ask you to complete in the privacy of your home. We will proceed through a series of steps, at a pace that is comfortable for both of you, to enrich your sexual life together. The exercises will be enjoyable and, given all the positive things you have going for you, I am optimistic that these exercises will help to make your sexual experiences more rewarding for you both.

"Does this plan make sense to you both?"

This sample formulation illustrates how we try to integrate biological, psychological, and social factors for a particular case. The steps involved in presenting a formulation include the following:

- Review the presenting problem, including normalizing the problem and educating the patient/couple as you go.
- Review the patient's/couple's strengths in the biological, psychological, and social domains.
- Identify the factors that appear to be responsible for the problem's development and maintenance; this is the core of the formulation.
- Invite feedback from the patient/couple regarding your formulation, including additional information that confirms or challenges it. Be careful not to encourage a debate on the matter, and acknowledge that

the formulation is meant to serve as a heuristic guide rather than an exact factual account.

- Outline the specific treatment components for addressing the causal factors, especially the maintaining factors associated with the dysfunction.

In general, we find that this approach gives the patients confidence that you have considered all possibilities, and that you are not just providing a "packaged" treatment program. Instead, this approach makes clear to patients that a specialized, customized treatment is adopted.

Special Challenges to Assessment

The assessment process is not without its pitfalls, potholes, and problems. We have already alluded to the technical skills, costs, and some obstacles to conducting a state-of-the-science assessment. We now turn our attention to more prosaic challenges to the assessment process.

The Uncooperative Partner

In a small number of our cases, a patient will enter therapy without the full cooperation of his or her partner. Some of these patients have partners who are reported to be shy but cooperative; in other cases, the partner believes that the problem is the patient's and refuses to participate. This always presents a difficult situation and one in which you can never be sure whether you have all the pertinent facts. To help an uncooperative partner become engaged in therapy, you can suggest talking to the partner by phone. If he or she still refuses, then you can suggest reading material that is pertinent to the problem.

Crucial components of therapeutic change (e.g., communicating effectively, cognitive restructuring, and dispelling blame) can almost never be achieved when one partner refuses to participate. This is especially true when the uncooperative partner is purported to be angry and blaming. You can, of course, offer some therapeutic benefit to the participating patient by providing etiological explanations and information, clearing up misunderstandings, putting the problem in perspective, and outlining strategies for change. However, you must also describe the limitations of therapy and try not to shift blame or fuel anger toward the absent partner. The end result of therapy is often a patient who has an improved understanding of the problem and feels better about him- or herself but still has a dysfunctional relationship with his or her partner.

Gay, Lesbian, and Bisexual Patients

Single gay, lesbian, and bisexual (GLB) patients or couples can usually be assessed in the same way that we suggest for heterosexual patients or couples. GLB patients who are comfortable with their sexual orientation are likely to present with sexual dysfunction concerns similar to those of heterosexual patients.

There are several therapeutic issues that can cause unique distress for GLB patients. First, GLB patients who do not yet accept or feel comfortable with their sexual orientation may benefit from preliminary work dealing with common issues such as various forms of discrimination, internalized homophobia, and self-damaging behavior (e.g., alcohol or other drug abuse; Shires & Miller, 1998). Second, GLB patients must navigate a less well-structured and patterned sexual world. The stereotypical gender and sexual roles that are normative may make less sense to them than they do for the heterosexual majority on whom such norms are based (Behrendt & George, 1995; Fassinger & Morrow, 1995). Third, in the United States, gay and bisexual men have been more likely to be infected with HIV; this raises concerns about mourning previous partners, secondary prevention, access to health care, and related issues. Although HIV is a threat to all sexually active people, regardless of their sexual orientation, the epidemiology of HIV in the United States (and most of the developed world) reveals that gay men have been disproportionately affected.

Because we cannot provide either a comprehensive review of GLB issues, or specialized coverage of the clinical approaches that have proven most effective, we recommend further reading for therapists who intend to work extensively with GLB patients (e.g., Behrendt & George, 1995; Coleman & Rosser, 1996; Fassinger & Morrow, 1995; Friedman & Downey, 1994; Herbert, 1996). As a final point, we wish to emphasize that if you are heterosexual and are uncomfortable treating GLB patients, then you should refer such patients to another therapist. Also, if a GLB patient is uncomfortable with you, their therapist, being heterosexual, then a referral to a GLB therapist may also be a good idea. We would be inclined to discuss patients' concerns but would, in the end, accept patients' preferences.

Single Patients without Partners

Patients without partners who are experiencing sexual dysfunction problems may require a few special considerations; in general, however, most of what has been discussed is applicable to these patients. It is common for a single patient to enter therapy after having experienced a "sexual failure." For men, this may have been an experience of premature ejaculation or erection failure, whereas for women this is likely to have been vaginismus, dyspareunia, or loss of desire. Regardless of the nature of the problem, single patients are likely to enter therapy with low self-esteem, sexual insecurities, and avoidance of social interactions. We try to be sensitive to these likely areas of concern and spend more time in identifying barriers that may impede social interactions.

Some single patients offer to bring in a casual partner to help with the therapy process. Our general approach is to allow a partner to participate only if there is a genuine commitment. The reason for this is to protect the patient, because assessment and therapy require the revelation and open discussion of vulnerabilities and intimacies that the patient may later regret having discussed. We have had some occasions when married patients offered to bring in lovers rather than their marriage partners. This situation presents obvious ethical concerns. We counsel patients on the pros and cons of legal separation and divorce. If a patient chooses to take no action, then the limitations and value of therapy must be fully discussed with the patient. Further suggestions regarding the treatment of single patients is provide by McCarthy (1992).

Patients Who Are Abusing Alcohol or Other Drugs

A great deal has been written about both the physical and psychological impact of chronic alcoholism on sexual functioning (O'Farrell, 1990; Wilson, 1981). It is well documented that alcoholic men and women experience a high prevalence of sexual problems (e.g., Jensen, 1984; Klassen & Wilsnack, 1986; O'Farrell, 1990; Tan, Johnson, Lambie, Vijayasenan, & Whiteside, 1984). Male alcoholics are susceptible to low desire and erectile dysfunction, whereas female alcoholics are at increased risk for low desire, orgasmic dysfunction, and vaginismus.

Although it is tempting to try to help patients with substance use disorders to improve their sexual functioning, we have learned that this is extremely difficult. We advise that you not treat the sexual problem if problem drinking or drug use is ongoing. Substance abusers should be referred for substance abuse treatment before sex therapy is attempted.

Concluding Comments

The assessment procedure necessary for accurate diagnosis of sexual dysfunction has continued to become more complex in recent years. We now understand that most sexual problems present with an interplay of medical and psychosocial factors, and demand a wide range of expert diagnostic input. This can be an expensive and, at times, a long process; we look forward to more streamlining in the future especially, because psychological and medical cooperation has grown stronger.

A comprehensive assessment interview cannot be separated from therapy. Within the assessment process, a patient's attitudes are often challenged, new information is learned, and misunderstandings are corrected. By asking patients about various factors that influence their sexual response, you are helping them to view the sexual problem as a state rather than as an unchangeable trait. This conceptualization is important to restore optimism to the patient and to his or her partner. Similarly therapeutic is the reduction or removal of blame for the sexual problem. Assessment solicits information from each partner; thus it helps redirect blame and guilt, and focuses the couple's energies on solving problems. Assessment also facilitates the breakdown of barriers to communication. This process is begun during the assessment, because the patient is asked to discuss details of his or her own sexual behavior and details of his or her partner's sexual behavior. Clients observe you, the therapist, discussing sexual matters in an open and nonthreatening manner, and this discussion models effective communication.

Thus, through the assessment process, couples are exposed to an appropriate communication style and are encouraged to discuss sexual matters in a constructive rather than a destructive or avoidant manner. It is not surprising that many couples report positive change in their attitudes, and in some cases, in actual sexual behavior, following assessment, before therapy proper begins.

7

Psychosocial Approaches to Treatment

Although misunderstandings about sex therapy remain, they have been reduced considerably in the age of Viagra. With very prominent, tasteful, and sensitive ads about sexual dysfunction now appearing daily on television and with numerous websites available for information on sex problems and sex therapy, the general public's understanding and acceptance of sexual dysfunction as a common and legitimate concern has increased greatly. Along with this increased understanding and acceptance has been knowledge of treatment options, including sex therapy. Our patients are more sophisticated now in their understanding of treatment options than were our patients 10 years ago. We have had no patients in recent years ask about sex surrogates as part of therapy, and with so much attention focused on sexual misconduct and inappropriate boundary crossing, we believe that the general public no longer wonders if sex therapy might include sex with the therapist. (We acknowledge that some providers still use "body-work" assistants [e.g., Apfelbaum, 2000], but this practice is rarer now than previously.)

Evidence for the Effectiveness of Sex Therapy

Early evidence for the efficacy of sex therapy came from the writings of Masters and Johnson (1970). Although quite encouraging, their methods were weak and did not provide the level of evidence that we currently require. However, within the past 30 years, there have a number of evaluations of psychosocially oriented sex therapy. For example, Hawton, Catalan, and Fagg (1992) studied outcome and prognostic factors in 36 couples who entered sex therapy because of the male partner's erectile dysfunction. The assessment and treatment approach was quite similar to that described in this book. It was based on the sensate focus approach described by Masters and Johnson (1970) but administered by a single therapist (rather than with cotherapists) during weekly (rather than daily) sessions. Treatment began after individual interviews with each member of the couple, followed by a conjoint interview, during which a formulation was presented. Homework assignments began with nongenital sensate focus and progressed to genital sensate focus, then to genital containment, and eventually to full sexual intercourse.

Two-thirds of the patients completed the treatment, with noncompletion associated with lower SES, the female partner having a history of psychiatric treatment, poorer motivation of the male partner, poor communication in the general relationship, and less sexual pleasure experienced by the female. Treatment success was achieved in 69% of the patients, with positive results being associated with better pretreatment communication and general sexual adjustment, especially the female partner's interest and enjoyment of sex, absence of a positive psychiatric history in the female partner, and a couple's early engagement in homework assignments.

Using a larger sample of 365 married couples, Sarwer and Durlak (1997) reported the results of a field trial of behavioral sex therapy. The couples had presented with a range of sexual dysfunctions at an outpatient sexual dysfunction clinic. Individual and conjoint assessments were completed prior to the interventions, which targeted performance anxiety, distraction from erotic cues, and deficits in sexual and interpersonal skills. Treatment components included education, communication skills training, and sensate focus exercises delivered during weekly sessions. The results indicated that outcomes for 65% of the couples was judged as successful, and there were very few dropouts (< 2%). Outcomes did not vary significantly as a function of diagnoses, gender, or a history of sexual abuse. It was interesting that the strongest predictor of successful treatment was the amount of sensate focus completed in the last week of treatment. These results indicated that behavioral sex therapy is effective in real-world clinical settings.

Heiman and Meston (1997) provided a comprehensive review of the research literature, examining a wide range of treatments for each of the dysfunctions discussed in this book. They concluded their impressive review by stating that "empirically validated psychological treatments for several dysfunctions exist, 'well established' in the case of primary anorgasmia in women, and erectile failure in men, and 'probably efficacious' for secondary anorgasmia and, perhaps, vaginismus in women and premature ejaculation in men" (p. 186). The evidence for the treatment of HSDD, sexual aversions, dyspareunia, and delayed orgasm in men is less convincing. Their review provides a useful summary of current knowledge and allows therapists to be more confident in applying the techniques we are advocating for achieving positive outcome.

It is possible to identify linkages between likely etiological explanations and indicated treatments based on our reading of the literature and clinical experiences. Thus, in Tables 7.1 through 7.4, we list the varieties of sexual dysfunctions, along with possible etiologies and treatments. The tables present each disorder for males and females, with consideration of whether the disorder is acquired or lifelong and generalized or specific. The listings of possible etiologies and treatments are not meant to be exhaustive but rather are representative of the most common or probable. Etiologies and treatments should not be assumed to be singular explanations. In most cases, there exist multiple etiologies and several treatment options. The connection in the tables between an etiology and a treatment means that for that etiology, the treatment listed is the most likely. Terms such as "medical," "surgery," or "psychotherapy" assume the most appropriate intervention for the problem within these treatment modalities.

In the remainder of this chapter, we describe the processes of sex therapy by clarifying what is actually done. This chapter covers general strategies for approaching any sexual dysfunction problem, as well as details of specific techniques.

An Overview of Sex Therapy

In spite of increased patient knowledge and sophistication regarding sex therapy, we still advise sex therapists to explain the content and process of therapy to each new patient. Patients appear to be put at ease and greatly appreciate an organized statement regarding what sex therapy will include and how a programmatic approach will be followed.

The outline presented in Chapter 6 for conducting a comprehensive assessment interview applies to the therapy as well. Thus, we recommend that you make assumptions, set goals, attend to process issues, and follow a planned structure. We develop each of these recommendations below.

Assumptions

As in the case of assessment, it is helpful to begin therapy with a set of assumptions. These assumptions are educated guesses (i.e., hypotheses) that you make in order to facilitate efficient and effective progress. Some helpful assumptions that may prepare you for common problems are as follows:

- The patient has a narrow definition of sex (e.g., "sex = intercourse"); he or she will focus on performance as a marker of success.
- The patient has stereotyped views of masculine and feminine sex roles; these views will interfere with the assimilation of new information.
- The patient does not understand the ingredients conducive to sexual arousal (e.g., favorable times to have sex, interfering factors).
- The patient has a pattern of avoidance of sexual interactions; as a result, he or she may unintentionally sabotage therapy.

By making these assumptions in advance, you will be prepared for potential pitfalls in the therapeutic process and increase the likelihood of success. We appreciate that some readers may find setting assumptions inappropriate, perhaps because this might suggest that we do not listen to what our patients bring to therapy. This is an important point to address. We believe that one can go too far in setting assumptions and encourage caution here. However, we also believe that most clinicians tend to have assumptions, and we simply urge you to make these more explicit and consistent with clinical experience. Of course, if the assumptions prove to be inaccurate, you must adjust your approach. We set up our assumptions such that, in most cases, an inaccurate assumption indicates a therapeutic gain.

Goals

In our view, the primary goal of therapy should be to create or restore mutual sexual comfort and satisfaction. More specific goals should be established only after the completion of a comprehensive assessment. We have found that patients often enter therapy with very specific goals, but that after the assessment, new goals need to be established. For example, a couple with severe communication problems may enter therapy with the goal of having the female partner experience coital orgasm. This goal, established by the couple, is not likely to be reached as long as angry conflict exists between the partners. It is your task as the therapist to help the couple to understand the psychological as well as the mechanical factors that contribute to satisfactory arousal and sexual enjoyment; in so doing, new goals are established.

New goals must be presented to the couple in such a way that the partners understand that in order to reach their goals, they must first work on preliminary goals. Moreover, it is important for the couple to understand that achieving these preliminary goals may cause discomfort. We encourage patients to conceptualize these preliminary goals as "stepping stones" or "building a foundation." Finally, and very importantly, goals should be discussed openly with the couple.

As a therapist, you need to be careful not to establish goals that increase performance anxiety. For example, goals such as "increasing erection firm-ness," "producing orgasm," or "controlling ejaculation" may actually exacer-bate the problem, especially if performance anxiety is inhibiting the response. If such performance-related outcomes do occur, they should be looked upon as pleasant side effects, secondary to achievement of the goal of increasing mutual pleasure.

Process

Many important interpersonal and interactive nuances can occur during ther-apy. Although these are not part of the planned therapy program, they can be crucial to therapy success. Factors such as your appearance, the appear-ance of your office, and your educational credentials may be important to a patient. Being responsive to patient requests for information and returning phone calls promptly also facilitate a positive rapport. These factors are present in any therapeutic interaction and are not the special domain of sex therapy.

Sex therapy brings with it its own set of important process issues. The discussion of sensitive and potentially embarrassing material requires special sensitivity. It is common for a patient to say, "I have never told this to anyone else before." Your reaction to such information is crucial and can either en-courage or discourage further discussion. As noted in Chapter 6, we have had patients say, "I tried to tell this to my doctor, but he appeared so uncomfort-able that I couldn't discuss it." You can encourage further discussion by ac-knowledging that the patient may find it difficult to discuss sexual topics, by reassuring the patient of your experience in dealing with sexual problems, and by remaining poised and calm, even if your patient(s) reveal information or sexual behavior that strikes you as bizarre (this does happen!).

Careful attention should also be paid to the development of therapist–patient feelings (i.e., transference and countertransference). Keep in mind that intimate discussion about sexual issues with a caring therapist may set the stage for sexual fantasies and attractions. As a therapist, you must be aware of the potentially seductive nature of the therapy process (especially with a single patient) and avoid the personalization of the therapist–patient relationship. If you suspect that the patient is behaving in a seductive manner, then the ther-apy should address this issue. If you feel attracted to your patient or find your-self behaving in a seductive manner, you should consult with a colleague im-mediately. Ask him or her to help you to assess the magnitude of the problem and to devise a strategy for working through this "countertransference." The colleague may encourage you to discuss the problem with your patient or to refer the patient to another therapist. We wish to make it clear that, from our perspective (and that of many professional organizations, we might add), sexual intimacy between a patient and therapist is unacceptable and cannot be justified under any circumstances.

If you are working alone (i.e., without a cotherapist) with heterosexual couples, you must avoid the appearance of taking sides. A couple will often make the assumption that a therapist is aligned with the same-gender patient. This issue should be discussed at the beginning of therapy, and throughout therapy as needed, to counteract such assumptions. We attempt to identify and repeat almost every session the issues that each partner has to work on independently (e.g., making more positive statements to his or her partner) as well as the issues that the couple has to work on together (e.g., setting aside time for communication or sensate focus). With this strategy, each partner should not feel that only he or she is the focus of change.

Structure and Content

The next consideration in sex therapy is the structure and content of therapy itself. As noted in Chapter 6, therapy begins during the assessment, when key target problems are identified. So, for example, if relationship issues are of sufficient magnitude to interfere with progress, these must be treated first. If relationship issues are not destructive or interfering, then sex therapy can begin. From our perspective, therapy can be construed as having three stages:

STAGE I

The first stage of sex therapy usually focuses on some or all of the following goals: acquiring knowledge, negotiating sexual differences, identifying desired sexual behaviors (and approaches to sex), and acknowledging performance anxiety. Depending on the extent of a couple's or individual's problems, this first stage of therapy may include anywhere from one to several session(s). Basically, Stage I therapy is focused on ensuring that proper knowledge, goals, and motivation exist to proceed with a focused, sex therapy approach.

STAGE II

The second stage of therapy involves the active work on more specific sexual goals identified during Stage I. This may include, for example, practicing new approaches and behaviors to reduce performance anxiety, using fantasy training to increase arousal, and practicing communication to reduce misunderstanding and express sexual desires. Cognitive approaches to improve maladaptive beliefs also occur during this stage.

STAGE III

The third stage of therapy involves reviewing treatment process and outcomes (to consolidate gains and achieve a sense of accomplishment), and planning for treatment generalization and relapse prevention. Stage III should begin when Stage II programs appear to be successful and moving along with only minimal therapist guidance. We begin this stage with a review of how the sexual problem developed, what the couple or individual was experiencing at the beginning of therapy, what goals were established, and what goals were achieved. Next, we discuss anticipated pitfalls in the future (that might lead to a recurrence of problems) and a review of the strategy to deal with such problems.

SPACING OF SESSIONS AND LENGTH OF THERAPY

Our general approach to most sexual dysfunction problems is to space sessions at weekly intervals. When possible, we will see patients at a more accelerated pace during the initial assessment. During therapy, however, our experience suggests that weekly sessions allow time for homework practice and reflection without losing continuity. The spacing of sessions should be reevaluated regularly to determine whether a different schedule will better serve the couple, for whatever reason, without disrupting the flow of therapy. If a couple or individual is very compliant in following therapy instructions, then spacing sessions every 2, 3, or even 4 weeks is possible once progress has been established. When sessions are spaced apart by more than a few weeks, instructions can be given that will allow for phone contact and even emergency sessions if needed. Most of our patients have been able to reach therapy goals successfully within 15 sessions.

This outline contains the elements of a comprehensive approach to sex therapy, but it is only a heuristic guide. It is always necessary to customize the treatment plan you develop to the needs of a patient or couple. In the next section, we provide details of several therapeutic procedures that are often useful when treating several sexual dysfunction problems.

General Techniques of Sex Therapy

There are several procedures that tend to be therapeutically useful for most sexual dysfunctions. In the next section, we discuss five of these: sensate focus, education, stimulus control, cognitive restructuring, and communication training.

Sensate Focus

Just as the interview serves as the cornerstone of sex assessment, sensate focus serves as the cornerstone for sex therapy. The sensate focus approach and procedures were initially developed by Masters and Johnson (1970), and can be used to address a number of aspects of improving an individual's or couple's sexual behavior. Thirty years later, we still find ourselves introducing this approach into a majority of cases we treat. Couples and individuals readily understand and appreciate this approach when it is explained adequately and tailored to their needs. We still find that many patients have attempted variations of sensate focus on their own or at the suggestion of their medical doctor or friends, but without success. The usual difficulty is performance pressure, even if a couple agrees not to perform! To avoid creating a demand for sexual performance is harder than it sounds and, in the back of most individuals' minds lingers the private thought that "if this works, I am going to go for it."

Under the guidance of a therapist, a strict adherence to the principles and purpose of sensate focus can more likely be followed. The therapist helps to keep couples on track and adjust procedures as needed.

PRINCIPLES

The first and most important principle of sensate focus involves helping the patient or couple to develop a heightened awareness of, and to focus on, sensations rather than performance—thus, "sensate focus." By doing this, a person or couple reduces anxiety by striving toward something that is immediately achievable (i.e., to enjoy touching), rather than striving toward a goal (e.g., erection, orgasm, controlled ejaculation) that may not be achievable; the latter increases the risk of "failure" and embarrassment. For some patients, we find it helpful to frame this principle as "Zen and the art of lovemaking," or "being in the here and now," or "enjoying the trip rather than focusing on the destination," or related metaphors. Most (but not all!) of our patients get the concept.

Second, sensate focus involves a structured but flexible approach to therapy. It is structured in that patients are given explicit instructions for intimacy; if these instructions are followed, the patients/partners will gradually regain confidence in themselves and in their relationship. Although it is structured in the sense that couples know what is expected of them, sensate focus is very flexible in that it can be accommodated to any couple's unique circumstances. It is critical that, as a therapist, you accommodate the procedures (described later) to the specific needs of your patients.

Third, sensate focus is a gradual approach to change. It is anticipated that change will take time, and there is no effort to rush ahead. Theoretically, the procedure of breaking down a complex behavior into smaller steps may be seen as a form of operant shaping, because an individual will gain a sense of accomplishment or self-efficacy through modest but attainable "successes" (Bandura, 1997); this may also be conceptualized as an *in vivo* desensitization procedure when anxiety reduction is the goal.

One example of this gradual success principle is that patients discontinue intercourse in the early stages of therapy, so that they can relearn the "basics" of being affectionate, receiving pleasure, and so on. For some patients, intercourse will not be reintroduced into their sexual repertoire for weeks or even months! The gradual approach can be off-putting to some because it can seem slow, especially in a culture that emphasizes speed—on the internet, in the microwave kitchen, and with "instant everything." Thus, special care is needed in explaining the importance of this gradual approach to patients.

Fourth, sensate focus therapy and home exercises need to be conducted in a shared and nonthreatening environment. As therapist, you need to attend to both partners in a couple to be sure that the exercises are proceeding at a nonthreatening pace.

You should be mindful of the principles behind sensate focus as you proceed. The procedures outlined below, and in other sources, are not intended to be followed in a cookbook-type fashion. Rather, they are offered as a heuristic guide and should only be followed as long as they are consistent with the spirit of the principles just outlined.

PROCEDURES

The actual procedures of sensate focus involve encouraging partners to approach intimate physical and emotional involvement with each other in a gradual, nonthreatening manner. The general operating procedure involves homework, which encourages the couple to engage in sexually related exercises, and ongoing therapy sessions, which are used to discuss the exercises, emotions triggered by these exercises, problems, and so forth.

Homework involves the provision of explicit instructions to the patients; these instructions require practice of some exercises outside of the therapeutic sessions. It is made clear to the patients that the homework will be reviewed and modified (as necessary) at each session. The homework exercises can be broken down into four "steps," which are typically followed in a sequential fashion, but there are no absolutes here. The decision whether each step should be included, and how much time should be devoted to each, requires your clinical judgment.

The first step of sensate focus typically includes "nongenital pleasuring" (i.e., touching) while both partners are dressed in comfortable clothing. The least threatening behaviors may include back rubs or holding hands. Variations in the amount of clothing worn, the length of sessions, who initiates, the types of behaviors participated in, and the frequency of sessions should all be discussed in the therapy sessions before a couple goes home to practice. The partners should begin their physical involvement at a level that is acceptable to both.

Because many couples will find this to be a somewhat slow and indirect method (to say the least), you must emphasize right from the start that (1) they are going through a necessary process in order to address their long-term goal, but that (2) the short-term goal is to focus on sensations and not performance. Discuss with each couple the mechanics of the approach, including structured versus unstructured approach, frequency, potentially interfering factors, and anticipation of any problems.

Even if you give what you believe to be a clear explanation of the nonperformance aspects of sensate focus, some patients will miss the point! So we try to be particularly explicit and remind patients: "The next time you have a therapy session, I will not ask you about erections or orgasms; what I will ask you about is your ability to concentrate on receiving and giving pleasure, and your ability to enjoy what you are doing." We repeat this message because most couples are performance-oriented (i.e., they focus on erection and orgasm); unless they are disabused of this notion, they will retain performance criteria during the sensate focus exercises.

At this point, you might also discuss with the patient or couple the concept of performance anxiety. This should include exposing "all-or-none" thinking (e.g., "sex = intercourse") and other factors that interfere with enjoyable sex. The application of sensate focus cannot proceed unless the partners understand this concept, acknowledge that it applies to them, and appreciate the need for a different approach in thinking and behavior.

The second step, typically, will involve "genital pleasuring." During this phase of therapy, partners are encouraged to extend gentle touching to the genitals and breasts. Partners are encouraged to caress each other, in turn, in a way that is pleasurable. As before, the couple should be discouraged from focusing on performance-related goals (i.e., erection, orgasm). As the therapy progresses through sensate focus, you should review factors that facilitate or inhibit goals. Discussing these factors with the partners in a nonjudgmental way can help them feel more in control of their own progress and less like pupils in a classroom.

Once a couple becomes comfortable with genital touching and is ready to resume sexual intercourse, we find it necessary to emphasize that even sexual intercourse can be broken down into several behaviors. Thus, we might encourage some couples to engage in "containment without thrusting"; that is, the receptive partner (i.e., the woman in heterosexual couples) permits penetration and controls all aspects of this exercise. For example, the depth of penetration and the amount of time spent on penetration can be varied. Again, we encourage flexibility and variation in order to remove pressure associated with a couple's tendency to think in "all-or-none" terms.

A common problem with this stage of sensate focus is that therapists rigidly adhere to the proscription on intercourse (Lipsius, 1987). If employed mechanically, proscription of intercourse can lead to loss of erotic feelings, loss of spontaneity, unnecessary frustration, and increased resistance. Our approach to the proscription issue is to discuss with the couple all of the potential benefits and liabilities of proscription, and to point out that the couple is working on a process that will build for the future. Pressure to ensure that a couple adheres to a proscription is dependent to a large degree on clinical judgment.

In our view, a proscriptive approach may be warranted under certain circumstances, for example: (1) if a couple is very stressed by "sexual performance," (2) when there are a lot of interfering performance-oriented thoughts, or (3) if the couple has avoided all physical contact. On the other hand, couples who have not approached sexual relations so rigidly or with such intense emotional reactions may benefit from a general understanding of the purpose of sensate focus, but with a more relaxed attitude toward proscription.

The final step of sensate focus proper includes thrusting and intercourse. Again, it is usually a good idea to encourage the receptive partner to initiate the movement, and for movements to be slow and gradual. As always, the couple is encouraged to focus on the sensations associated with intercourse, and not to be concerned about orgasm. Urge partners to experiment with different positions and discouraged them from relying on the same position(s) they have used prior to therapy.

These are the general procedures that constitute what is commonly referred to as sensate focus. Several authorities have elaborated the basics provided here (e.g., Hawton, 1985; Kaplan, 1974; Masters & Johnson, 1970); you may want to consult these references once you have worked comfortably with the steps as described earlier. At this point, however, we want to identify some of the potential problems that you are likely to encounter.

PITFALLS OF SENSATE FOCUS

The sensate focus has potential applications and benefits for many of the problems encountered by sex therapists. Unfortunately, the procedures are often misunderstood and misapplied. It is not unusual for couples to enter therapy and report that they had tried to "abstain from sex" or "just fondle" and this did not work. Recently, a couple enrolled in therapy for the purpose of dealing with erectile difficulties. In response to a question about past therapy, the man explained that they had previously participated in sex therapy and had tried sensate focus. The approach used was "not to have sex for a 2-week period."

The couple had no understanding of the purpose of the procedure or the guide-lines for their behavior. They left their previous therapy very dissatisfied.

We often encounter variations of the misapplication of sensate focus. It is a very simplistic procedure on the surface and a very effective strategy, but it is easily misapplied and misunderstood by both therapist and patient. McCarthy (1985) has pointed out a number of the common mistakes in the use of sensate focus homework assignments.

The most common mistake that therapists make is not explaining the de-tails of the procedure and not engaging the couple in the decision-making pro-cess of the application. This often results in noncompliance. A second com-mon mistake is demanding performance as part of the procedure (e.g., "The next step in the procedure is to stimulate your partner in the genital area to the point of orgasm."). This type of statement may increase performance anxiety, especially in a vulnerable person. It would be preferable to state, "You have done well so far in concentrating on your sensations and feelings as you and your partner stimulate each other. Thus far you have included genital caress-ing. What do you feel the next step should be?" This approach allows a variety of responses without an anticipation of sexual failure or pressure. One addi-tional mistake some therapists make involves premature termination of the sensate focus approach when a couple is noncompliant or encounters difficul-ties. Premature termination only serves to reinforce avoidance. Difficulties should be discussed at length, and barriers to progress should be identified and removed. Generally, we allow 3 weeks of noncompliance before changing procedures.

Another opportunity for disaster presents itself when therapy moves into the area of "homework procedures." At this time, there exists a potential con-flict between being natural and unstructured, and being mechanistic and struc-tured. Most couples and individuals express a preference to approach home-work assignments in a "natural, unstructured" manner. With this approach, you describe the procedures involved and the principles behind the proce-dures, but leave it up to the couple to schedule other details, such as the fre-quency and times for "practice." Although you may feel intuitively that this is preferred strategy, you can expect couples to return to therapy without having carried out the assignment! The reason for this is that, all too often, there is a long history of sexual avoidance; thus, the individual or couple cannot get started without raising anxiety levels unacceptably high.

Thus, we usually explain the pros and cons of structured versus unstruc-tured strategies before providing homework exercises. The couple can then choose a strategy and, in so doing, can be fully aware of the potential for non-compliance. At times, a patient may "try out" a certain strategy and, upon fail-ure, may adopt a different approach. In addition to exploring the issue of structured versus unstructured practice, you should explore other potential ob-stacles to carrying out therapy procedures—for example, children or other family living in the house, work schedules, medical concerns, and travel plans. Once these potential obstacles are identified, and solutions generated, then the rationale and details of homework can begin.

BENEFITS OF SENSATE FOCUS

There are many benefits that may result from the sensate focus approach. New behaviors may be learned, along with new approaches to sexual interactions. We have dealt with couples who have had very narrow approaches to sex. It is not unusual, for example, for a couple to report that they engage in no touching behavior at all. They may kiss once, then have intercourse! We have even encountered couples who view foreplay as "something that kids do." For such a couple, sensate focus offers a structured opportunity to challenge established habits that may be restricting pleasure and causing sex problems.

Sensate focus may also help to change patients' perception of their partners. A common problem we run into is that many men approach sexual intimacy with intercourse and orgasm as the only goals. In a heterosexual couple, the female partner may begin to see herself as an object of her partner's pleasure and not as a companion who is loved. The sensate focus procedure can help partners to focus on each other with mutual affection rather than as sexual toys or objects of arousal.

Sensate focus also offers an opportunity for individuals to learn to communicate with their partners about sexual pleasures and preferences. It is not at all unusual to encounter couples who have been married for many years and yet have no idea what the partner likes or dislikes about sex. As mentioned in Chapter 6, the Index of Dyadic Heterosexual Preferences (Purnine et al., 1996) can be a useful assessment device, but it can also be used in therapy as a conversation starter about differential preferences in a couple. We have sometimes had partners complete the measure twice: once for themselves, and a second time for their partner. When asking them to complete it for their partner, we suggest: "Indicate how much you believe that your partner would agree or disagree that the statement is true for him or her; that is, respond to each item as you think your partner would respond—how he or she would actually like things to be in relations with you." Then, we compare the perceived preferences for each partner to the actual preferences and discuss discrepancies. This can be quite enlightening to the couple, and can help to introduce the importance of communication.

As the therapist, you should point out to your patients undertaking sensate focus that this procedure offers an opportunity to give feedback to one another. The feedback, if delivered during the throes of sex, does not have to be in the form of carefully expressed verbal statements (!) but may be delivered with expressions (e.g., "ooh," "ahh," or the like), or by moving a partner's hand to a preferred spot. Afterwards, partners can compliment one another, for example, "I really liked it when you. . . . "

Sensate focus can also be quite diagnostic. Difficulties that emerge during sensate focus often carry important information about a couple's other problems. These other problems often cannot be addressed through sensate focus itself, but the exercises can elicit such concerns that might otherwise go unnoticed.

CONCLUDING COMMENTS

Sensate focus should be viewed as one part of a total treatment approach; *it is not a complete therapy in itself.* Thus, communication issues, faulty attitudes that interfere with sexual enjoyment, and nonsexual marital conflicts are examples of therapy concerns that may be dealt with concomitantly with sensate focus. Sensate focus is a procedure that has multiple benefits and can be used as part of a treatment program for every category of sexual dysfunction problems.

Education

Education (i.e., providing information) may be the most common component of sex therapy. Conceptual models (Fisher & Fisher, 1992, 1998) often recognize that sexual health interventions must provide information, motivation, and behavior skills training if they are to be effective. Such models make explicit what most clinicians know: that knowledge is necessary, but it is not sufficient for behavior change.

Information can help to correct myths and to reverse misunderstandings that adversely affect sexual functioning. For example, the belief that foreplay is for kids, or that intercourse is the only true form of sex, can be devastating to a middle-aged or elderly male and his partner. Similarly, the belief that the erection must appear first (i.e., before sexual activity) in order to signal sexual interest and desire can limit a person's sexual opportunities. The net effect of these beliefs is that a male who does not obtain an erection prior to a sexual interaction will not participate in sex. We have known men and women who have avoided sexual interactions for years, partly because of an adherence to these beliefs.

Education about the normal changes in male and female functioning due to aging can be used to support the important and "normal" role of foreplay in adult sexual activity. The belief that foreplay is for kids may have had its origin in the common Italian practice of *carezza*; this term refers to the nonintercourse sexual play activity practiced by Italian youths. In some parts of Italy it is still a ceremony to "show the sheets" to the bridegroom's father after the wedding night. Blood must appear on the sheets to reassure the father that his son has married a virgin.

Zilbergeld (1999) and Wincze and Barlow (1997a) list other common myths to which you may want to address:

- Men should not have (or at least not express) certain feelings.
- In sex, as elsewhere, it's performance that counts.
- The man must take charge of and orchestrate sex.
- A man always wants and is ready to have sex.
- All physical contact must lead to sex.
- A man should be able to last all night.
- Too much masturbation is bad.
- When you have a sex partner, you shouldn't need or want to masturbate.
- Sex equals intercourse.
- Sex requires an erection.
- Good sex is a linear progression of increasing excitement terminated only by orgasm.
- Fantasizing about something else means I am not happy with my current partner.

You can also help your patients by debunking myths. In this regard, we are reminded of one patient who entered therapy with very low self-esteem. The source of his distress was a "problem" with premature ejaculation: He confessed that he usually reached orgasm within 15 minutes of vaginal penetration. He was surprised, to say the least, to learn that the period from intromission to orgasm among American men typically ranges from 2 to 7 minutes (Kinsey et al., 1948).

It is clear that you can serve a valuable role by just providing accurate information. For example, giving an elderly woman information about the use of vaginal lubricants (e.g., Replens, Astaglide, Today, and Lubrin or Condom Mate suppositories) may alleviate her pain during intercourse. Also, pointing out to a couple or individual that biological factors may play a role in the dysfunction can relieve guilt or blame. It is likewise helpful to provide correct information about anatomy and physiology, as well as normative sexual behavior. To aid with education about anatomy, you may want to purchase medical illustration books or even three-dimensional anatomical models that can be found in most medical school bookstores.

Given that education can be therapeutic, the question arises: How can you best educate a patient in the context of sex therapy? Here, as elsewhere, we advise flexibility. Some patients like to read and request suggestions for reading material. Indeed, there is evidence from 12 controlled studies that bibliotherapy for sexual dysfunctions (especially the directed practice approach to orgasmic disorders) can be quite effective (van Lankveld, 1998). The effect tends to diminish over time, however, but this is also true of face-to-face therapy.

Not everyone likes to read. Other patients prefer to ask questions during therapy. Still others will be reluctant to ask for information directly; for these patients, you will need to take advantage of naturally occurring opportunities to given an impromptu "lecture."

Fortunately, for patients who like to read, there are many excellent books available. We can recommend several titles (see below), and we encourage you to develop your own reading list. You may want to purchase several copies of your favorite guides and have them available to loan out (be careful, however; you may not get them back!). Alternatively, you might identify one or two local bookstores and encourage patients to purchase their own copies. In any event, we advise that you read any book that you recommend to a patient and be prepared to discuss its contents during the sessions.

RECOMMENDED READINGS FOR PATIENTS

There are several excellent books that we can recommend for you to share with your patients.

Gottman, J., Notarius, C., Gonso, J., & Markman, H. (1979). *A couple's guide to communication.* Champaign, IL: Research Press.

Gottman, J. M., & Silver, N. (1999). *The seven principles for making marriage work.* New York: Crown.

Heiman, J. R., & LoPiccolo, J. (1988). *Becoming orgasmic: A sexual and personal growth program for women* (rev. ed.). New York: Prentice-Hall.

Kaplan, H. S. (1989). *How to overcome premature ejaculation.* New York: Brunner/Mazel.

Kilmann, P. R., & Mills, K. H. (1983). *All about sex therapy.* New York: Plenum.

McCarthy, B. (1998). *Male sexual awareness: Increasing sexual satisfaction* (rev. and updated ed.). New York: Carroll & Graf.

McCarthy, B., & McCarthy, E. (1993). *Sexual awareness: Enhancing sexual pleasure.* New York: Carroll & Graf.

McCarthy, B., & McCarthy, E. (1998). *Couple sexual awareness.* New York: Carroll & Graf.

Michael, R. T., Gagnon, J. H., Laumann, E. O., & Kolata, G. (1994). *Sex in America: A definitive survey.* Boston: Little, Brown.

Schover, L. R. (1997). *Sexuality and fertility after cancer.* New York: Wiley.

Tannen, D. (1990). *You just don't understand: Women and men in conversation.* New York: Morrow.

Wincze, J. P., & Barlow, D. H. (1997). *Enhancing sexuality: A problem solving approach.* San Antonio, TX: Psychological Corp.

Zilbergeld, B. (1999). *The new male sexuality* (rev. ed.). New York: Bantam.

A critically important area in which you should be prepared to address your patients' concerns and questions involves HIV and other STDs. Although there are several excellent books available for patients (e.g., Kalichman, 1998), information regarding HIV transmission, screening, testing, and treatment is also widely available through state and federal health organizations. You can call your local or state Health Department for free brochures to have available for patients. There are many telephone hotlines available for you or patients to call for the latest information, and the resources available online are absolutely amazing. Some of our favorite websites are *www.caps.ucsf.edu*, *www.hopkins-aids.edu*, *www.positive.org*, and *www.cdc.gov*.

Creating a Conducive Environment for Sex: Stimulus Control and Scheduling

We have encountered many situations in which individuals present with complaints of sexual dysfunction yet are attempting to have sex under adverse conditions. It is often perplexing to us that men and women expect to function sexually when there are circumstances present that are decidedly nonsexual. Consider the following example: A 50-year-old, single, male patient had recently lost both of his parents, whom he had lived with all of his life. He was coming to therapy because, since the death of his parents, he had started dating a woman to whom he was very attracted. However, he had experienced erectile dysfunction when the relationship became intimate. When questioned about his sexual experiences with his new girlfriend, it was learned that he was able to have "successful" sexual intercourse with her in her apartment on one occasion but failed three times when sex was attempted at "his place." Further questioning revealed that sex at his place was always attempted in his deceased parents' bedroom. To make matters worse, in this room was a three-foot crucifix over his parents' bed, with portraits of his mother and father on either side. He explained his choice of location for his "lovemaking" as having a bigger and more comfortable bed. He had not identified his lovemaking circumstances as a source of interference, although, once explored, he acknowledged that he might have felt guilty.

Stimulus control refers to efforts to establish a pleasant, relaxing, and erotic environment that is conducive to sexual expression and minimizes interfering circumstances. Although the aforementioned case presents very obvious interfering stimuli, sex can also be interfered with under less obvious conditions. Time pressures and the presence of disruptive stimuli, such as having kids who are light sleepers in an adjacent bedroom, are often cited. Because individual differences are so great when it comes to identifying erotic as well as nonerotic conditions, it is the task of the therapist to help a couple be aware that conditions for sex matter. Once this concept is understood (which may include challenging some long-standing beliefs such as "love conquers all" or "a willing partner is all that is needed"), then the therapist can help a couple identify the conditions that facilitate (or hinder) sexual comfort.

Another myth that emerges commonly is that of "spontaneous sex." What we mean by this is the view expressed by patients that sex should not have to be planned, and should just occur spontaneously if people are in love. Many patients forget all the planning that went into "spontaneous" sexual expression during courtship. We sometimes encourage patients to schedule couple time, and to plan for it with as much effort as they might for any other special event in their lives. We remind them that anticipation often fuels desire, and that there is nothing wrong with setting a "date" with a long-standing partner.

For couples who balk at the idea of "planned" sex, remind them that you are addressing the need to plan and prioritize the opportunities for sex, and not the sex itself.

Cognitive Restructuring

Two forms of cognitive restructuring can be helpful: (1) challenging negative attitudes and (2) reducing interfering thoughts.

CHALLENGING NEGATIVE ATTITUDES

Exposing and helping a patient to change negative attitudes is a complex therapeutic task. One of the differences between a myth (or misunderstanding) and a negative attitude is that the latter is held onto tenaciously, despite compelling data to the contrary. For example, a woman may have very negative feelings toward men and believe that men cannot be trusted. This attitude may be the result of having a harsh or rejecting father, or a history of sexual abuse, or a previous relationship in which the woman's partner was unfaithful. In this woman's current relationship, she may interpret her partner's erectile failure as evidence of being unfaithful. If it is clear that the erection failure is due to other factors, it may take considerable therapeutic effort to address her general negative and untrusting attitude toward men, which was established previously and has, perhaps, helped her to avoid hurtful relationships.

Similarly, a male may have a negative and untrusting attitude toward women; for example, he may perceive all women as manipulative and only seeking a partner for safety, security, or status. His "lack of desire" may be a reflection of his fear of making a commitment and being manipulated. Again, you may have to address this attitude before working directly on the sexual problem. In all cases, this should be approached with caution—a patient may be very defensive and have a great deal invested in holding onto a negative belief. You may have to deal with such issues in individual therapy before couple therapy can proceed.

REDUCING INTERFERING THOUGHTS

Sometimes you will need to help a patient reduce intrusive images or thoughts that are interfering with sexual enjoyment. A man who worries about the firmness of his erection, or one who worries about having sex with a new partner in the bed that he and his deceased wife shared for 30 years, may experience interfering thoughts and sexual problems. The presenting problem may be loss of erection, loss of desire, or delayed ejaculation, but the source of the problem is the interfering thoughts. Similarly, a woman who worries about her sick child, or about professional responsibilities and commitments, may lose her sexual desire or be unable to achieve orgasm. It is always intriguing that despite the obvious presence of interfering thoughts, many patients ignore or dismiss such thoughts as contributors to sexual difficulties; instead, they focus on the perception of their own, or their partner's, inadequacy.

To deal with interfering thoughts, you must first help the patient identify the presence of such thoughts. Once such thoughts are identified, and it is agreed that interfering thoughts do occur in association with sexual behavior, then you must help the patient reduce the occurrence of such thoughts. It may be helpful to encourage patients to focus on erotic thoughts during sexual activity. For example, focusing on body parts or a sequence of sexual activities is usually more conducive to arousal. However, you should be prepared for such suggestions to lead to discussions about whether it is "normal" or "healthy" to fantasize about sex (or about sex with another partner) during actual sexual activity. Some patients feel very strongly that fantasizing is tantamount to cheating on one's partner. (We are reminded of the scandal caused by then-President's Jimmy Carter's disclosure in *Playboy* that he had sinned in his heart because he was attracted to women in addition to his wife.) Obviously, such discussions have to be approached with a great deal of care and sensitivity. We also find it helpful to have patients read the chapter on sexual fantasies in McCarthy's (1998) book, *Male Sexual Awareness: Increasing Sexual Satisfaction.*

It may also be helpful to a patient to suggest compartmentalizing thoughts. Specific times during the day should be set aside to focus on worrying and problem solving; other times should be set aside for pleasant and sexual thoughts. Putting such categories of thoughts on schedule may help teach a patient to eliminate negative thinking during sexual time periods.

Negative beliefs and interfering thoughts can present impediments to sexual expression and enjoyment. In some cases, it will be possible to address these cognitive difficulties as a part of the sex therapy itself. In other cases, however, more intensive cognitive restructuring may be needed, usually in the context of individual therapy. Because cognitive therapy techniques and process can be quite involved and quite useful, we recommend that you familiarize yourself with more detailed accounts of these methods (e.g., Beck, 1976; Ellis, 1962; Meichenbaum, 1977).

Communication Training

Communication problems are encountered frequently when dealing with sexual dysfunction. We have developed a handout for patients that serves as both an assessment tool and a therapeutic guide. The handout is 10 pages long and describes common couples' communication problems and provides suggestions about how to overcome these problems. The typical problems in communication include the following:

Off beam: Partners start to discuss one problem and drift into another.

Mind reading: Partners guess the meaning of each other's statements because they think they know each other so well.

"Kitchen sink": Partners start discussing one problem and bring in every other problem.

"Yes, but": Each partner listens but continues to think that the other is wrong.

Cross-complaining: Each response contains a new complaint.

Standoff: Partners tend to repeat the same argument over and over, without progress or resolution.

We have found it both time saving and helpful to hand out the communication pamphlet to all couples, regardless of whether they present with obvious communication problems. We typically instruct patients to read the handout independently (we give one to each partner) and ask them to check off the patterns that might apply to their relationship. We then discuss the various areas of communication difficulties, often with examples from the couple's own experiences. It is very important for you to establish from the beginning that the review of the examples is designed to look at the process of communication and not to illustrate or determine who was right or wrong.

As the therapist, you should serve as a model of good communication during all sessions. This is achieved by listening actively, displaying empathy, asking patients to express themselves clearly, and other such social and communication skills. In addition, you should continually look for improvement in communication skills and point these out to a couple when they occur. It is helpful for you to inform the couple that, throughout the therapy, communication skills will be monitored continually and addressed when appropriate. If this is stated at the outset, an individual will not feel picked on when a communication issue is raised.

In some cases, sexual dysfunction problems cannot be addressed until communication improves. In such cases, we often point out that sexual expression is a specific form of communication and that it will be enhanced by focusing on general communication training.

Much has been written on communication training for couples; for further training, we recommend the excellent works by Beck (1988) and Gottman, Notarius, Gonso, and Markman (1976). The latter is also useful as a guide for patients.

Safer Sex Guidelines

There is no such thing as "safe" sex. To be sexually active is to take a chance of becoming infected with a STD, such as HIV. There have been many recent reports of infection with HIV among monogamous women (Gangakhedkar et al., 1997). Just because one partner is monogamous does not guarantee that his or her partner has been.

Throughout the therapy process, you can help patients to minimize their risk for STDs by using "safer" sexual practices. For many (especially newer) couples, it is wise to advise that they both get tested for HIV before engaging in unprotected insertive (oral, vaginal, or anal) intercourse. If the couple is committed to mutual monogamy, safer sexual practices can be discontinued once testing determines that neither partner is infected. In single patients, we suggest that they minimize the number of sexual partners, avoid high-risk activities (e.g., unprotected vaginal or anal intercourse), avoid partners who engage in high-risk activities, remain alert to any symptoms of infection, use condoms in any situation other than a long-term, mutually monogamous relationship (preferably after mutual HIV counseling and testing), wash with soap and water after every sexual contact, and urinate after intercourse.

More detailed strategies for enhancing motivation for safer sexual practices and increasing condom negotiation skills are widely available (e.g., Carey et al., 1997, 2000; Kelly, 1995; Kalichman, 1998).

Procedures for Specific Problems

In the previous section, we described several generic therapeutic procedures as well as circumstances that are encountered in the treatment of almost all sexual problems. In the next section, we describe more focused procedures for specific problems.

Desire Disorders

Low sexual desire in men or women can be related to a number of biological and psychosocial factors, as identified in Chapter 2. During the assessment, you must first determine whether the problem is situational (i.e., specific to the patient's current situation and functioning) or generalized (i.e., a more pervasive problem). A careful assessment should identify potential etiological factors. For example, is low desire due to a long-standing negative attitude toward sex? And, if so, is this due to sexual trauma or poor parental role modeling? Is low sexual desire due to one particular partner or set of circumstances, or is the low desire present in all sexual situations? In addition, low desire may be the end product of severe performance anxiety, in which a person has selectively ignored and avoided erotic stimuli because of the threat such stimuli pose. As always, a careful assessment is essential to formulating the problem and planning treatment.

GENERALIZED DESIRE DISORDERS

When low desire is a product of long-standing attitudinal and experiential factors, therapy must focus on processing the source and reaction to the important background influences. The patient must develop an understanding of the influences on his or her low desire. Because insight alone rarely results in any positive change, increasing desire may only develop following positive sexual experiences. However, even when positive experiences are encouraged through sensate focus, long-standing desire problems can be resistant to change. Exposure to erotic and/or masturbatory training may also be used in resistant cases to promote change.

Before discussing the use of erotica in the treatment of desire disorders, a small discussion is necessary to define terms and clarify our position. When we use the term "erotica," we are referring to the depiction of consensual sexual relations, whereas the term "pornography" refers to the depiction of coercive sexual relations. Our position regarding the use of erotica is similar to that articulated by the Sexuality Information and Education Council of the United States (SIECUS):

> When sensitively used in a manner appropriate to the viewer's age and developmental level, sexually explicit visual, printed, or on-line materials can be valuable educational or personal aids, helping to reduce ignorance and confusion and contributing to a wholesome concept of sexuality. However, the use of violence, exploitation, or degradation, or the portrayal of children in sexually explicit materials is reprehensible. Minors should be legally protected from all forms of sexual exploitation. (available from the SIECUS website at *www.siecus.org*)

We appreciate, however, that some readers and patients may have different views on the use of erotica, and we respect their views. We also appreciate that it can be challenging to find erotica that is healthy in the way that it depicts less powerful persons, including women.

Use of erotic materials should proceed only after a thorough discussion with the patient. Objections to pornography, particularly the objectification and degradation of women, should be addressed, so that there are no barriers to accepting and experiencing erotic materials positively. When you are confi-

TABLE 7.1. Likely Etiologies and Possible Treatments for the Desire Phase Dysfunctions

Dysfunction	Likely etiologies	Possible treatments
Male hypoactive sexual desire (acquired/generalized)	*Medical:* 1. Low testosterone (various causes) 2. Elevated prolactin (pituitary adenoma) 3. Medication side effect 4. Medical disease *Psychosocial:* 1. Depression 2. Worry/anxiety 3. Sexual trauma 4. Sexual performance anxiety	1. Testosterone (endocrinologist, urologist) 2. Dopamine agonist (endocrinologist) 3. Medication adjustment 4. Medical 1. Psychotherapy 2. Psychotherapy 3. Trauma therapy 4. Sensate focus, erotic exposure, fantasy training
Male hypoactive sexual desire (acquired/specific)	*Medical:* None *Psychosocial:* 1. Partner conflict 2. Sexual performance anxiety 3. Environmental interference	 1. Couple therapy 2. Sensate focus 3. Environmental adjustments, erotic exposure, fantasy training
Male hypoactive sexual desire (lifelong/generalized)	*Medical:* 1. Endocrine problem 2. Other chronic illness *Psychosocial:* 1. Sexual trauma 2. Negative sex messages 3. Low self-esteem or poor self image	1. Medical/endocrinologist 2. Medical 1. Trauma therapy 2. Educational information, sensate focus, desensitization 3. Psychotherapy, sensate focus, desensitization
Male hypoactive sexual desire (lifelong/specific)	*Medical:* None *Psychosocial:* 1. Sexual orientation dysphoria/confusion 2. Sexual trauma 3. Negative sex messages	 1. Psychotherapy/counseling 2. Trauma therapy 3. Educational information, sensate focus, desensitization

TABLE 7.1. (continued)

Dysfunction	Likely etiologies	Possible treatments
Female hypoactive sexual desire (acquired/generalized)	*Medical:* 1. Hormone imbalance 2. Medication side effect 3. Medical disease *Psychosocial:* 1. Depression 2. Worry/anxiety 3. Sexual trauma	 1. Hormone therapy 2. Medication adjustment 3. Medical 1. Psychotherapy 2. Psychotherapy 3. Trauma therapy
Female hypoactive sexual desire (acquired/specific)	*Medical:* None *Psychosocial:* 1. Partner conflict 2. Environmental interference	 1. Couple therapy 2. Environmental adjustments, erotic exposure, fantasy training
Female hypoactive sexual desire (lifelong/generalized)	*Medical:* Chronic disease *Psychosocial:* 1. Sexual trauma 2. Negative sex messages 3. Low self-esteem or poor self-image	 Medical 1. Trauma therapy 2. Educational information, sensate focus, desensitization 3. Psychotherapy, sensate focus, desensitization
Female hypoactive sexual desire (lifelong/specific)	*Medical:* None *Psychosocial:* 1. Sexual orientation dysphoria/confusion 2. Sexual trauma 3. Negative sex messages	 1. Psychotherapy/counseling 2. Trauma therapy 3. Educational information, sensate focus, desensitization
Male sexual aversion (acquired/generalized)	*Medical:* Physical trauma or disease to genitals *Psychosocial:* Sexual trauma	 Medical (urologist), psychotherapy Trauma therapy, desensitization, sensate focus

(continued)

TABLE 7.1. (*continued*)

Dysfunction	Likely etiologies	Possible treatments
Male sexual aversion (acquired/specific)	*Medical:* None	
	Psychosocial: Sexual trauma	Trauma therapy, desensitization, sensate focus
Male sexual aversion (lifelong/generalized)	*Medical:* Congenital genital deformity, body deformity	Medical/surgical, psychotherapy
	Psychosocial: 1. Sexual trauma	1. Trauma therapy
	2. Negative sex messages	2. Educational information, sensate focus, desensitization
	3. Body image	3. Psychotherapy
Male sexual aversion (lifelong/specific)	*Medical:* None	
	Psychosocial: 1. Sexual trauma	1. Trauma therapy, desensitization, sensate focus
	2. Sexual orientation or gender dysphoria, confusion	2. Psychotherapy, counseling
	3. Negative sex messages	3. Educational information, sensate focus, desensitization
Female sexual aversion (acquired/generalized)	*Medical:* Physical trauma or disease to genitals or breasts	Medical, psychotherapy
	Psychosocial: Sexual trauma	Trauma therapy, desensitization, sensate focus
Female sexual aversion (acquired/specific)	*Medical:* None *Psychosocial:* Sexual trauma	Trauma therapy, desensitization, sensate focus

TABLE 7.1. (*continued*)

Dysfunction	Likely etiologies	Possible treatments
Female sexual aversion (lifelong/generalized)	*Medical:* Congenital genital/body deformity	Medical/surgical, psychotherapy
	Psychosocial: 1. Sexual trauma	1. Trauma therapy
	2. Negative sex messages	2. Educational information, sensate focus, desensitization
	3. Low self-esteem or poor self-image	3. Psychotherapy, desensitization, sensate focus
Female sexual aversion (lifelong/specific)	*Medical:* None	
	Psychosocial: 1. Sexual trauma	1. Trauma therapy, desensitization, sensate focus
	2. Sexual orientation or gender dysphoria, confusion	2. Psychotherapy, counseling
	3. Negative sex messages	3. Educational information, sensate focus, desensitization

dent that your patient can use erotic materials without negative objections, then the nature and details of exposure should be discussed. Use of erotica should be approached as a sexual experience, paying attention to mood, setting, and other important ingredients of a satisfying encounter. It is also crucial to advise the patient to view erotica without being a movie or literary critic! We have had patients return after viewing erotica and comment on the poor cinematography. Developing your own library of materials that you have previewed, so that you can make knowledgeable recommendations to patients, is a good idea.

Masturbation training with fantasy must be approached in a fashion similar to the use of erotica. Negative attitudes must be explored first, then detailed attention must be paid to maximizing a positive sexual experience. We do not assume that a patient knows how to masturbate. For example, we had a patient who reported to us a lack of success in attempting to masturbate. When he was asked how he masturbated, he reported that he masturbated with his hand open so that his palm rubbed against the underside of his penis. In addition, he reported putting honey on his penis as a "lubricant." He thought he read somewhere that honey was a good lubricant. Another male patient who reported difficulty with masturbation put his penis between the palms of both hands; he then rubbed his penis back and forth, much in a way a Boy Scout might try to start a fire with a stick! Specific instructions with pictures helped both of these patients to learn how to masturbate successfully.

Masturbation training can help some patients to become more sensitive to the conditions necessary for a positive sexual experience. In patients who lack desire and sexual confidence, masturbation training can lead to positive experiences that build both desire and confidence. Although most experts agree that there are no right or wrong techniques of masturbation, there are techniques that are less efficient (such as the open-handed technique described earlier) or potentially harmful (masturbating with a vacuum hose). The therapist should encourage patients to explore the best techniques and conditions for masturbation.

SITUATIONAL DESIRE DISORDER

When low desire is linked only to a current partner or circumstance, change can usually be achieved more easily. Solving the problems with the current partner or circumstance must be addressed first; then a return of sexual desire can be facilitated. If increase in desire does not follow a resolution of current problems, then sensate focus, exposure to erotica, or masturbatory training may be helpful.

An often overlooked circumstantial cause of low desire is habituation. This is especially true of couples in long-term relationships, who always approach sex in the same fashion. With a recent case, we initially had some difficulty in pinpointing the cause. The partners seemed to be very compatible and communicated effectively. They also were relatively liberal and approached sex with a lot of creativity and variety. During one session, which the male partner attended alone because his partner was on a business trip, he was asked whether there was anything he had not discussed previously: "You know what really bugs me? She goes around the house completely nude all the time. As soon as she comes home from work, she strips down to nothing and stays that way all night. She also never wears underwear and even tells our friends about this. She tells me that I'm a prude if I'm not naked and, if we sit next to each other, I have to hold her hand or else she will touch my penis. I hate that! Also, she never closes the bathroom door when she goes to the bathroom and comes right in when I'm going. There is no privacy whatsoever in our home."

As an example of habituating to a partner, this case was somewhat extreme; however, we often encounter couples who are completely open with their toileting behavior and nudity. Although there is nothing wrong with this, it is not uncommon for such openness to lead to habituation. Theoretically, this is consistent with Stoller's (1975) view that novelty and risk are the motivating forces behind sexual desire and arousal. Thus, whether couples are very conservative or very liberal in their approach to sexual relations, habituation can be a factor contributing to low desire.

Another common expression of low desire occurs in partners with different levels of desire. Initially, this difference may be masked because one partner (usually the less desirous) accommodates the other. Over time, however, some resentment develops and the problem surfaces. In such couples, it is common for the less desirous partner to be labeled as the "patient." As it turns out, however, there is simply a discrepancy between a relatively low-desire partner and a relatively high-desire partner. In such couples, you can expect communication and problem-solving skills to be poor; these will require attention before the partners can begin to negotiate a sexual pattern that is mutually acceptable and satisfying.

We have also found that low sexual desire often results from partner incompatibility. Partners, whether married or unmarried, homosexual or heterosexual, may have difficulty in articulating to each other that there is little or no sexual attraction between them. There may be unresolved anger or incompatibility just because a couple has "grown apart." At any rate, it is common for the role of the therapist to shift to helping a couple identify and deal with their incompatibility separately from the sexual issue. The focus on low desire may have been the catalyst that brought a couple to therapy to deal with their ambivalent feelings toward each other. In separate interviews with each partner, you can sometimes elicit descriptions and feelings of desire for other persons or circumstances separate from the partner. Your role may then be to help the partners accept their low desire for each other and to put this information into perspective. This does not necessarily result in separation for a couple and may even lead to a peaceful acceptance of their situation.

Male Erectile Disorder

More is now known about erectile disorder than any other sexual dysfunction. Thanks to multidisciplinary research, we now have an extensive understanding of the biopsychosocial mechanisms of erectile dysfunction. The medical aspects of treatment are addressed in the following chapter. It should be pointed out, however, that even in cases where significant biomedical factors have been identified, psychological factors may also be present and must be considered in treatment.

Once a comprehensive assessment has been completed and the relative contributions of biomedical and psychosocial factors can be determined, a specific treatment program can be designed. As the therapist, you should also be aware that erection problems may have evolved as a result of premature ejaculation, delayed ejaculation, or lack of desire. All of these potential problem areas should be explored thoroughly, along with the comprehensive medical and psychosocial assessment of the erection problem.

Treatment may include any of the treatment approaches we have already discussed. Indeed, the approach to treating erectile disorder has in the past relied largely upon relationship approaches, particularly sensate focus. Given current knowledge, we are now more sensitive to including in our treatment approach consideration of the individual factors discussed in Chapter 3 and outlined by Barlow (1986).

Many males who experience erectile difficulties become very upset with themselves and fear embarrassment in front of their partners. In heterosexual males, fears of homosexuality may emerge; that is, heterosexual men often interpret difficulty in obtaining or maintaining an erection as a sign that they are gay. In both homosexual and heterosexual males, erection difficulties raise fears regarding masculinity. Regardless of the precipitating factors, many cases of erectile disorder are maintained by interfering thoughts that may precede and occur during sexual relations. As we explain to our patients, these interfering thoughts are not erotic or sexy; moreover, they decrease arousal and inhibit erection. In a sexually functional man, thoughts that precede and occur during sexual relations usually focus on his partner's or his own body parts, seductive behaviors, and anticipations of arousal and pleasure. In contrast, the dysfunctional male is preoccupied with worries regarding the firmness of his erection; images of his partner being disappointed, angry, or even ridiculing; and distinct feelings of anxiety, embarrassment, and depression.

The treatment of erectile disorder must address the interfering thoughts by helping the man to "restructure" his thoughts, that is, to focus on sexually facilitating thoughts rather than on sexually inhibiting ones. The term "performance anxiety" (Masters & Johnson, 1970) is often applied to the dysfunctional thinking, but focusing on anxiety can be misleading. Several studies have shown that anxiety can actually facilitate rather than inhibit arousal (Barlow et al., 1983; Hoon, Wincze, & Hoon, 1977; Wolchik et al., 1980). Indeed, Barlow (1986, 1988) has presented compelling evidence that the thought processes of dysfunctional males contribute to the erectile differences.

One way to help the patient to refocus his thinking onto more positive thoughts is to have him recall his thought content during past satisfying sexual experiences. This usually sensitizes him to the types of thoughts on which he might concentrate. If he has difficulty remembering positive sexual thoughts, you may wish to help him with "typical" helpful thoughts. This is an instance where exposure to erotic literature or videotapes may be helpful.

Once your patient is able to identify the positive sexual thinking process, he is ready for sensate focus. You can now establish the goal (during sensate focus) of thinking positively about sex rather than achieving or maintaining an

TABLE 7.2. Likely Etiologies and Possible Treatments
for the Arousal Phase Dysfunctions

Dysfunction	Likely etiologies	Possible treatments
Male erectile disorder (acquired/generalized)	*Medical:*	
	1. Diabetes, neurological disease, vascular disease	1. Medical, Viagra, implant, vasoactive injection
	2. Low testosterone	2. Testosterone therapy (urologist or endocrinologist)
	3. Elevated prolactin	3. Dopamine agonist (endocrinologist)
	4. Other medical disease	4. Medical, Viagra
	Psychosocial:	
	1. Performance anxiety	1. Sensate focus
	2. Depression	2. Psychotherapy
	3. Worry/anxiety	3. Psychotherapy
	4. Sexual trauma	4. Trauma therapy
Male erectile disorder (acquired/specific)	*Medical:* None	
	Psychosocial:	
	1. Partner conflict	1. Couple therapy, sensate focus
	2. Sexual orientation dysphoria/confusion	2. Psychotherapy, counseling, sensate focus
	3. Environmental interference	3. Environmental adjustment
Male erectile disorder (lifelong/generalized)	*Medical:*	
	1. Endocrine problem	1. Endocrine therapy
	2. Other chronic illness	2. Medical, Viagra, implant, vasoactive injection
	Psychosocial: Severe psychological disorder	Psychotherapy
Male erectile disorder (lifelong/specific)	*Medical:* None	
	Psychosocial:	
	1. Sexual trauma	1. Trauma therapy, Viagra
	2. Sexual orientation dysphoria/confusion	2. Psychotherapy/ counseling
	3. Negative sex messages	3. Educational information, sensate focus, desensitization

(continued)

TABLE 7.2. (*continued*)

Dysfunction	Likely etiologies	Possible treatments
Female sexual arousal (acquired/generalized)	*Medical:* 1. Menopausal	1. Hormone therapy, lubricant
	2. Other medical disease	2. Medical
	Psychosocial: 1. Performance anxiety	1. Sensate focus
	2. Depression	2. Psychotherapy
	3. Worry/Anxiety	3. Psychotherapy
Female sexual arousal (acquired/specific)	*Medical:* None	
	Psychosocial: 1. Partner conflict	1. Couple therapy, lubricant
	2. Environmental interference	2. Environmental adjustment, lubricant
Female sexual arousal (lifelong/generalized)	*Medical:* 1. Congenital endocrine problem	1. Endocrine therapy
	2. Other medical condition	2. Medical
	Psychosocial: 1. Sexual trauma	1. Trauma therapy
	2. Negative sex messages	2. Educational information, sensate focus, desensitization
Female sexual arousal (lifelong/specific)	*Medical:* None	
	Psychosocial: 1. Sexual trauma	1. Trauma therapy
	2. Sexual orientation dysphoria/confusion	2. Psychotherapy/ counseling
	3. Negative sex messages	3. Educational information, sensate focus, desensitization

erection. Remember, the patient is likely to focus on his erection and to report success or failure on this basis. Your job is to return his focus to erotic thoughts and images, not the erection.

Throughout treatment, you should monitor and attend to interfering thoughts, communication, conducive erotic environment, feelings of comfort, and good partner relationship. You should also help your patient to avoid performance-oriented approaches to sex by accepting a broad definition of sex; that is, the goal is to help the patient to see that sex is more than just intercourse; instead, sex involves a wide range of behaviors. We find the use of a menu analogy to be very helpful as a way to reduce performance pressure and to broaden the definition of sex. With this analogy, patients are told to conceptualize sex as a meal, and to pick and choose from the menu, depending upon their appetite and taste. Appetite and taste for sex may be expected to vary from occasion to occasion and person to person.

Even in cases where there is clearly a biomedical basis for the erectile problem, psychosocial issues should be considered in treatment. Negative, interfering thoughts (especially in long-standing problems) may be present in many cases of erectile disorder.

When a man's partner is involved in treatment, it is also important to consider his or her cognitions concerning the dysfunction. Just as the man with erectile difficulty harbors negative associations around this problem, so too, the partner is likely to have negative cognitions. Typical partner responses in homosexual as well as heterosexual couples may include the following:

"I'm no longer attractive."
"He doesn't love me anymore."
"He must be having an affair with someone else."
"He isn't trying; he doesn't want to have sex with me."

We always ask the partner what he or she thinks is the cause of the erectile problem. It is important to help to clear up possible misunderstandings before proceeding to an intervention, such as sensate focus exercises. If potential misunderstandings are not addressed, it is likely that they will arise again and sabotage treatment progress.

As with other dysfunctions, we assume that a couple is approaching sexual relations in a manner that may not be optimal for arousal to occur. On many occasions, we have encountered patients who do not kiss, touch, fondle, stroke, or hug prior to attempting intercourse; yet these patients expect an erection to emerge once they attempt intromission! Inquire about the details of the foreplay, as well as the erotic environment. Try to determine whether each partner is satisfied with what has been occurring.

The arrival of Viagra has had a major impact on the treatment of erectile dysfunction. Although details of the therapeutic use of Viagra will be discussed in Chapter 8, we wish to note here that Viagra can be helpful as an adjunct to the psychosocial therapeutic approach. We have had cases of men with psychogenic erectile disorder who have used Viagra on a frew occasions and, upon experiencing erections, have regained confidence. Subsequently, they have approached sexual relations more positively without using Viagra. It seems that just knowing that the Viagra works relieves a man of worry and allows him to disregard his performance anxiety. One might think of this as a type of sexual "safety net."

Female Orgasmic Disorder

Female orgasmic disorder is often experienced psychologically in a similar fashion to a man's experience of erectile disorder. In both conditions, performance anxiety can play a prominent role and maintain the problem regardless of the original cause. As in erectile disorder, worry about the outcome interferes with the sexual process and healthy functioning. And the harder one tries to achieve a sexual goal, whether it is erection or orgasm, the more unlikely that the goal will be achieved.

Female orgasmic disorder, a very frustrating dysfunction, can lead to a total avoidance of sexual relations. Because of the strong association with performance anxiety, sensate focus is often advised. In many cases, however, the suspected cause is a lack of sufficient erotic input, often associated with distracting and interfering thoughts. Directed use of masturbation with appropriate use of erotica is often helpful, especially in cases of primary anorgasmia. As in the case of other dysfunctions, it is necessary to conduct a detailed assessment to determine whether the problem has always existed (i.e., lifelong or generalized) or is associated with a current problem or condition (i.e., acquired or situational).

The book *Becoming Orgasmic* (Heiman & LoPiccolo, 1988) outlines in detail a program for helping women to learn to masturbate and to become orgasmic. This is a revised edition of a widely acclaimed earlier volume; it provides excellent information and its approach to the problem is considered state of the science. Research indicates that directed masturbation approaches are successful in at least 80% of cases with primary female orgasmic disorder (Heiman, 2000; LoPiccolo & Stock, 1986).

We have also found in many instances that female orgasmic disorder is associated with negative feelings toward sex (in general), oneself, or one's partner. With some patients, we have also encountered fears regarding fainting, losing control, or increased vulnerability. Rarely, in our experience, is the difficulty just a problem of poor sexual technique. In order to use a procedure such as masturbation training, you should first explore in detail whether negative cognitions and attitudes are present. It would be a strategic blunder to suggest masturbation training without first assessing the woman's and her partner's beliefs about the nature of the problem and the acceptability of masturbation. Once these feelings have been explored and both partners are comfortable, the physiology of orgasm should be explained and masturbation training initiated.

It is also important to explore a woman's expectations about orgasm to

TABLE 7.3. Likely Etiologies and Possible Treatments for the Orgasmic
Phase Dysfunctions

Dysfunction	Likely etiologies	Possible treatments
Male orgasmic (acquired/generalized)	*Medical:* 1. Substance abuse 2. Medication effect 3. Other medical	1. Substance abuse therapy 2. Medication adjustment 3. Medical
	Psychosocial: 1. Sexual trauma 2. Insufficient stimulation	1. Trauma therapy 2. Educational information, vibratory stimulation, lubrication, erotic exposure
	3. Performance anxiety 4. Unspecified psychological problems	3. Sensate focus 4. Psychotherapy
Male orgasmic (acquired/specific)	*Medical:* None	
	Psychosocial: 1. Partner conflict 2. Partner technique or solo technique	1. Couple therapy 2. Educational information
Male orgasmic (lifelong/generalized)	*Medical:* Congenital medical	Medical
	Psychosocial: 1. Unspecified psychological 2. Sexual orientation or gender dysphoria, confusion	1. Psychotherapy 2. Psychotherapy/counseling
Male orgasmic (lifelong/specific)	*Medical:* None	
	Psychosocial: 1. Sexual trauma 2. Negative sex messages	1. Trauma therapy 2. Educational information, sensate focus, desensitization
	3. Sexual orientation or gender dysphoria, confusion	3. Psychotherapy/counseling

(continued)

TABLE 7.3. (*continued*)

Dysfunction	Likely etiologies	Possible treatments
Premature ejaculation (acquired/generalized)	*Medical:* Unknown	Anafranil, Prozac, or Zoloft
	Psychosocial:	
	1. Performance anxiety	1. Sex therapy approach as outlined in this text
	2. Misinformation, poor technique	2. Educational information
Premature ejaculation (acquired/specific)	*Medical:* None	
	Psychosocial:	
	1. Couple conflict	1. Couple counseling, information
	2. Performance anxiety	2. Sex therapy as outlined in this text
Premature ejaculation (lifelong/generalized)	*Medical:*	
	1. Unknown	1. Anafranil, Prozac, or Zoloft
	2. Age related (under 35)	1. Educational information, Anafranil, Prozac, Zoloft
	Psychosocial:	
	1. Performance anxiety	1. Sex therapy as outlined in this text
	2. Misinformation, poor technique	2. Educational information
Premature ejaculation (lifelong/specific)	*Medical:* None	
	Psychosocial:	
	1. Performance anxiety	1. Sex therapy as outlined in this text
	2. Partner conflict	2. Educational information, couples therapy
	3. Misinformation, poor technique	3. Educational information
Female orgasmic (acquired/generalized)	*Medical:*	
	1. Disease process	1. Medical
	2. Substance abuse	2. Substance abuse therapy
	3. Medication side effect	3. Medication adjustment, vibratory stimulation

TABLE 7.3. (*continued*)

Dysfunction	Likely etiologies	Possible treatments
Female orgasmic (acquired/generalized, *cont.*)	*Psychosocial:*	
	1. Performance anxiety	1. Sensate focus, desensitization
	2. Sexual trauma	2. Trauma therapy
	3. Depression	3. Psychotherapy
	4. Worry/anxiety	4. Psychotherapy
Female orgasmic (acquired/specific)	*Medical:* None	
	Psychosocial:	
	1. Partner conflict	1. Couple therapy, information, sensate focus
	2. Poor partner technique	2. Educational information
	3. Environmental interference	3. Environmental adjustment
Female orgasmic (lifelong/generalized)	*Medical:* Various medical conditions	Medical
	Psychosocial:	
	1. Sexual trauma	1. Trauma therapy
	2. Negative sex messages	2. Educational information, sensate focus, desensitization
	3. Poor technique, lack of experience	3. Educational information, masturbation training, vibratory stimulation
Female orgasmic (lifelong/specific)	*Medical:* None	
	Psychosocial:	
	1. Sexual trauma	1. Trauma therapy
	2. Negative sex messages	2. Educational information, sensate focus, desensitization

ensure that they are realistic. Explaining that orgasm occurs on a continuum from mild to intense is often helpful. Some women we have treated have expected ground-shaking experiences every time and have dismissed mild rhythmic contractions as "not the real thing." Explaining the range of experiences helps to normalize a woman's sexual response and reduce worry.

Male Orgasmic Disorder

This disorder continues to be one of the most difficult to treat when there are no pharmacological or biological causal explanations. Because most men are easily orgasmic, it is unusual for a man to not experience orgasm when there is adequate sexual stimulation. The sexual stimulation can be sufficient to evoke an erection but apparently not sufficient to produce orgasm. Men presenting with male orgasmic disorder often give a history of low sex interest and/or negative sex messages. Additionally, there may be interfering factors such as not allowing sufficient time for creating a sexual mood. Such men may find success on a vacation but not at other times.

Therapy often needs to address the issue of creating a sexual mood through allowing sufficient time combined with increasing erotic input (fantasies, lubrication, vibrator, sex play). The use of a vibrator as an adjunct to other approaches is also often very helpful for treating inhibited delayed orgasm in men and women. Careful discussion about attitudes toward and techniques in using vibrators (i.e., avoid direct stimulation of the clitoris or glans because this could be too intense and painful), and where to buy vibrators (chain stores such as Wal-Mart, drugstores, adult sex shops and, of course, internet sites), should precede any prescription for use. As the therapist, you should present the idea of using a vibrator as exploratory and requiring practice (including trial and error) to benefit. The practice may be solo or in partnership and must occur in a stress-free and private environment.

Premature Ejaculation

Complaints of premature ejaculation are often associated with misunderstandings about sex and are also often "smoke screens" for relationship problems. Common misunderstandings include an unrealistic expectation about the length of time thrusting should last before ejaculation, and the belief that sex ends as soon as ejaculation occurs.

In many cases of premature ejaculation, we direct our initial discussion to the question, "Why do you have sex?" With this question (or a similar one), we try to elicit a man's hopes and goals when he has sex. After some thought, most men can generate quite a number of reasons. "To have pleasure" or "because it feels good" may be men's most common responses. We point out that people have sex for a variety of reasons: to experience pleasure, to express love and affection, to make up after an argument, to have children, to make oneself feel better, to please a partner, and so on. Moreover, the reasons may change from occasion to occasion. The goal of this general discussion is to impress upon our patients that pleasure or pleasuring, and all of the other reasons people have sex, are not dependent on the length of time between intromission and orgasm. Furthermore, the length of time a man "lasts" should be looked upon as but one small part of the whole sexual exchange. Indeed, the primary goal of our question and the ensuing discussion is to encourage the couple to focus on general pleasuring rather than orgasm. We encourage the partners to continue having intercourse even after ejaculation. We hasten to add, however, that this technique may be helpful for focusing a couple's attention on pleasure rather than orgasm, but it may not be desirable for couples practicing "safer sex"; that is, if a man does not withdraw after ejaculating, his condom may come off as detumescence begins. For men wearing condoms during sexual relations, the squeeze technique or stop–start procedure may be preferable.

Our purpose with this technique is to take the pressure off the timing of ejaculation and emphasize the total sexual relationship. This approach usually results in a couple's report of a more satisfying relationship. Interestingly, even though we do not focus on the length of time between intromission and ejaculation, this time interval does often increase.

A second question that we ask men experiencing premature ejaculation is "What do you believe is causing the problem?" As is the case with all sexual problems, the meaning attributed to the problem by each partner should be explored thoroughly. In some cases of premature ejaculation, the female partner may express anger because her sexual needs are going unmet. Similarly, some women may believe that men have more control over ejaculation than is truly the case; a woman may interpret her partner's "haste" as his way of being thoughtless or inconsiderate. However, we have yet to have a patient who can control his ejaculation so expertly that he can purposely reach orgasm quickly in order to hurt his partner's feelings. On the contrary, most men who seek treatment for premature ejaculation want desperately to increase their latency so that they can please their partners. They tend to be embarrassed and confused about their difficulty.

We want to point out, however, that a focus on premature ejaculation can be a distraction from the real problem. If the root cause is, for example, a distressed relationship, therapy directed at improving the relationship may also improve the premature ejaculation. When you believe that a couple has no sexual misunderstandings and has a compatible relationship, then the well-known "squeeze technique" can be applied (Masters & Johnson, 1970). The squeeze technique involves instructing the male to masturbate to a point that he feels would result in ejaculation if he continued. He should pause in the masturbation at this point and squeeze the head of his penis along the coronal ridge by placing his forefinger and middle finger on one side of his penis and his thumb opposite, on the other side. The squeeze should be firm and last about 10 seconds. By repeating this process several times before allowing ejaculation to occur, and by practicing this procedure over a number of sessions, the man may learn to better control his ejaculation.

Another procedure that is sometimes advised for controlling premature ejaculation is the "start–stop," or "pause," technique (Semans, 1956). This technique is the precursor to the squeeze technique. The couple is asked to practice foreplay and penile stimulation to the point prior to ejaculation. The male with premature ejaculation signals his partner when to stop, so that his arousal level can subside. Stimulation is then resumed after a pause, and the process is repeated at least three times before allowing ejaculation to occur. It is important to instruct the male to enjoy his sensations and to learn to identify the various levels of arousal that he experiences. Even though this technique has been around for 35 years, it is still considered a viable option that is used as one component of a total therapy approach. It should be noted that with both the squeeze and the stop–start technique, there is a danger of unwittingly reinforcing a performance-oriented message. These techniques should be used judiciously and only in cases in which a couple has embraced the philosophy of "whatever happens is OK."

As a final point, we should note that one of the side effects of the selective serotonin reuptake inhibitors (SSRIs), including such commonly prescribed medications as fluoxetine (Prozac), sertraline (Zoloft), and clomipramine (Anafranil), is delayed ejaculation. Thus, this particular side effect may be beneficial to men experiencing chronic premature ejaculation. The SSRIs seem to be helpful in cases of premature ejaculation (Kaplan, 1994; Balon, 1996; Segraves, Saran, Segraves, & Maguire, 1993; Metz et al., 1997).

When suggesting these techniques, whether pharmacological or behavioral, you should take care not to depict ejaculation control as a complete solution of a couple's problem. Ejaculation control should be viewed as part of, and not the totality of, satisfying sex.

Vaginismus and Dyspareunia

For both vaginismus and dyspareunia, a complete medical evaluation is advised to rule out any possible biomedical factors. The most common psychosocial explanation of vaginismus and dyspareunia is found in prior sexual trauma and negative sexual messages. Overcoming these problems often involves the complex task of reviewing and processing negative attitudes about sex. Once the patient is comfortable with a positive attitude toward sexual relations, then it is possible to initiate an *in vivo* desensitization procedure involving gradual insertion of a finger or dilator into the vaginal opening. It is probably more convenient, and easier for most women, to practice insertion using their own fingers. Some women, however, are more comfortable using a graduated set of dilators, perhaps because of phobic reactions to their genitals. The dilators may be obtained from a medical supply firm and come in graduated thicknesses.

The strategy should be thoroughly discussed and reviewed with a patient before actually suggesting it. It may be helpful to approach the topic by saying, "Some women who have difficulty with penetration have found that by practicing insertion very gradually, they can overcome the problem. How would you feel about the technique of practicing insertion while you are alone and in the complete privacy of your home?" Once a woman has agreed to try, you should explain that she (the patient) is in complete control of the procedures. It should be emphasized that the depth and length of time of penetration can be controlled and varied by the patient. The patient should approach this while bathing or while relaxing on her bed. She should start by inserting a finger or the narrowest dilator, and only when she is comfortable with inserting a dilator for a period of 5 minutes should she move on to the next size. A vaginal lubricant can be used. Over a number of sessions, she should work up to inserting two fingers or the largest dilator for a few minutes. Because some women will have strong objections to touching their genitals or masturbating, this exercise has to be put into perspective and distinguished from masturbation. It must also be emphasized that the purpose is desensitization, not arousal.

As a woman becomes more comfortable with insertion, her partner can be included in the procedure. Again, it should be emphasized that the woman must be in complete control of the procedure and that she can stop at any time. Moreover, the insertion process should be approached gradually, with partial penetration and withdrawal. This process is usually started with digital penetration; over a number of sessions, the couple moves toward penile insertion. Use of vaginal lubricants may be a useful addition to the insertion procedures.

Additional Considerations

Religious and Cultural Concerns

Occasionally you may encounter a patient who is in a bind because his or her religious or cultural beliefs clash with a more open approach to sex. For example, masturbation or even sensate focus may conflict with some religious teachings. You should, of course, always be sensitive to the possibility of such issues and never proceed with therapy until religious and culturally based beliefs related to sexual practice are explored thoroughly.

In a few cases, we have found that a patient's misinterpretation of a religious teaching has stood in the way of therapy. In such cases, it is helpful to

TABLE 7.4. Likely Etiologies and Possible Treatments for the Sexual Pain Disorders

Dysfunction	Likely etiologies	Possible treatments
Male pain (acquired/generalized)	*Medical:* 1. Peyronie's disease 2. Urinary tract 3. Genital injury *Psychosocial:* Somatization disorder, hypochondriasis	1. Surgical or medical treatment 2. Antibiotics 3. Urology Psychotherapy
Male pain (acquired/specific)	*Medical:* None *Psychosocial:* 1. Malingering, avoidance 2. Partner technique	 1. Psychotherapy 2. Educational information
Male pain (lifelong/generalized)	*Medical:* Congenital anatomical (stricture) *Psychosocial:* Somatization disorder	 Medical/surgical Psychotherapy
Male pain (lifelong/specific)	*Medical:* None *Psychosocial:* 1. Somatization disorder 2. Malingering, avoidance	 1. Psychotherapy 2. Psychotherapy
Female pain (acquired/generalized)	*Medical:* 1. Infection, STD 2. Endometriosis 3. Menopausal 4. Lesions, tumors *Psychosocial:* 1. Sexual trauma 2. General anxiety 3. Negative sex messages 4. Fear of pain	 1. Medical 2. Medical 3. Hormone therapy, lubricant 4. Medical 1. Trauma therapy 2. Psychotherapy 3. Educational information, sensate focus, desensitization 4. Sensate focus, gradual *in vivo* insertion

TABLE 7.4. (*continued*)

Dysfunction	Likely etiologies	Possible treatments
Female pain (acquired/specific)	*Medical:* None	
	Psychosocial:	
	1. Partner issues	1. Couple therapy, sensate focus
	2. Sexual trauma	2. Trauma therapy, sensate focus
	3. Environmental interference	3. Environmental adjustment
Female pain (lifelong/generalized)	*Medical:*	
	1. Congenital anatomical	1. Surgical
	2. Vulvitis	2. Medical
	3. Idiopathic body chemistry, neurological	3. Medical
	Psychosocial:	
	1. Sexual trauma	1. Trauma therapy, sensate focus
	2. Somatization disorder	2. Psychotherapy
	3. Negative sex messages	3. Educational information, sensate focus, gradual *in vivo* insertion
Female pain (lifelong/specific)	*Medical:* None	
	Psychosocial:	
	1. Sexual trauma	1. Trauma therapy, sensate focus
	2. Negative sex messages	2. Educational information, sensate focus, *in vivo* gradual insertion
Vaginismus (acquired/generalized)	*Medical:*	
	1. Lesions, tumors, genital trauma	1. Medical
	2. Sequelae to vaginal pain disorder	2. Medical

(*continued*)

TABLE 7.4. (*continued*)

Dysfunction	Likely etiologies	Possible treatments
Vaginismus (acquired/generalized, *cont.*)	*Psychosocial:* 1. Sexual trauma	1. Trauma therapy
	2. Sexual anxiety	2. Educational information, sensate focus, desensitization
	3. Fear of pain	3. Sensate focus, gradual *in vivo* insertion
Vaginismus (acquired/specific)	*Medical:* None	
	Psychosocial: 1. Partner issues	1. Couple therapy, sensate focus
	2. Sexual trauma	2. Trauma therapy, sensate focus
	3. Environmental interference	3. Environmental adjustment
Vaginismus (lifelong/generalized)	*Medical:* 1. Congenital, anatomical	1. Surgical
	2. Sequelae to vaginal pain disorder	2. Medical
	Psychosocial: 1. Sexual trauma	1. Trauma therapy, sensate focus
	2. Somatization disorder	2. Psychotherapy
	3. Negative sex messages	3. Educational information, sensate focus, gradual *in vivo* insertion
Female pain (lifelong/specific)	*Medical:* None	
	Psychosocial: 1. Sexual trauma	1. Trauma therapy, sensate focus
	2. Negative sex messages	2. Educational information, sensate focus, gradual *in vivo* insertion

refer the patient to an appropriate member of the clergy who can interpret the teaching and work in consultation with you.

Alcohol and Drug Abuse

Alcohol and drug abuse can adversely affect sexual functioning biologically. There can also be an adverse effect interpersonally and psychologically. We have found that it is not effective to work on sexual problems when there is an ongoing substance abuse problem. In almost all cases, the substance abuse problem must be treated first and be under control before a consistent program for sexual dysfunction can be implemented.

Other Psychological Disorders

It is not unusual for some of your patients to present with major psychological disorders. Individuals with personality disorders or neurotic disorders may be very challenging as you attempt to address their sexual concerns. Sometimes the psychological problems may be so overwhelming that a focus on the sexual issues is inappropriate or even impossible. Psychological testing and a careful psychosocial interview will help you to decide which problem is most important to address first. We have found that when psychological symptoms interfere with progress in a session, then the focus must switch to the treatment of the psychological disorder. We have conducted therapy by shifting our focus of attention depending on a patient's needs. Obviously, if such an approach interferes with progress in both areas, then a concentrated effort must be made to address the psychological problems until they are under control.

We have found that attempting to work with individuals manifesting organic brain syndrome is difficult and, for the most part, unsuccessful. Such patients may not be able to understand or focus on the important aspects of therapy. Individuals with symptoms of organic brain syndrome should undergo thorough neuropsychological testing. Consultation with a neuropsychologist will often give valuable information as to the capabilities of a patient to retain and process instructions and sexual information.

Typical Presenting Problems: Case Examples

Just as assessment is much more complex today than it was in the past and often requires a multidisciplinary effort, therapy for sexual problems has also increased in complexity and often must take into account other medical and psychological treatment issues. We believe it is a fitting conclusion to this chapter to briefly describe the presenting problems of four cases that we dealt with in a typical week, to illustrate the variety of problems a sex therapist may encounter.

Case 1

Mr. Reynolds is a 48-year-old gay man who works as an executive. He presented with a complaint of erectile dysfunction. He is now involved with a man who is 35 but feels sexually insecure. He is looking for a long-term relationship and believes that his partner of 6 months is also committed to a long-term relationship, but he is insecure because of their age difference. He wonders if Viagra would be helpful.

Case 2

Mr. and Mrs. Mouftan presented with complaints of male orgasmic disorder and infrequent sexual relations. They have been married for 10 years and are both successfully employed in middle-management positions. Mr. Mouftan works about 60 hours a week and, once at home, is busy working around the house or doing errands. Mr. and Mrs. Mouftan are both in their late 30s and would like to conceive a child. They are very happy with each other and will consider intrauterine insemination with the husband's sperm if sex therapy fails.

Case 3

Mr. and Mrs. Baum are in their mid-20s and have been unable to have intercourse in their 4 years of marriage. Mrs. Baum says she enjoys sex but is fearful of penetration. She was raised in what she describes as an "Old World" family. She was not allowed to date and lived with her parents until she graduated from college and got married.

Case 4

Mr. Sullivan is a veteran of the Vietnam war who suffers from chronic back pain and posttraumatic stress disorder. He and his wife have been married for 21 years and state that they love each other very much. However, they are both frustrated by Mr. Sullivan's erectile difficulties. Exogenous testosterone was prescribed by a urologist when below-normal levels of testosterone were detected. Although testosterone helped somewhat, getting adequate erections remain a problem most of the time and the couple requests treatment for this.

These four challenging cases are complex and require both medical knowledge and cultural- and sexual-orientation sensitivity. They illustrate the diversity of skills and training that today's therapists need.

8

Integrating Psychosocial and Biomedical Approaches

The most significant change in the treatment of sexual dysfunction in recent years has been the extensive use of Viagra to treat male erectile disorder. Many other pharmacological agents for the treatment of sexual dysfunction in men and women are currently undergoing clinical trials and can be expected to be made available (and marketed heavily) in the near future. With the advent of effective pharmacological agents for treatment of sexual dysfunction there is, surprisingly, an even greater need for the cooperative integration of medical and psychological approaches.

There has been a tremendous amount of publicity and advertisement surrounding Viagra. Indeed, when U.S. Senator and presidential candidate (Bob Dole) goes public with his erectile dysfunction, people notice. This increased media attention has brought an awareness and legitimization of sexual functioning concerns. Patients have been going in large numbers to their primary care physicians and family medicine physicians to obtain Viagra.

Although Viagra has been helpful for a large number of patients, physicians have discovered that it is not appropriate, nor is it effective, for all patients. Some patients are unable to take Viagra because they are taking nitrate-based medications. Others simply prefer a nonmedical solution in order to avoid unwanted side effects or the addition of a new medicine to their bathroom cabinet. Others experience upsetting side effects and discontinue the medication. Also, as has happened with other medicalized treatments, it may be possible to facilitate erections but, because of the lack of normally erotic cues, sex can still be frustrating and unfulfilling. When the focus is on the suc-

161

cess of the erection rather than on intimacy, arousal, and mutual pleasuring, the net result can be painful intercourse, intercourse with a delayed or disappointing orgasm, or other undesired consequences.

In short, no matter how effective a medical approach may be, there will still be a significant number of men and women who can benefit from additional help for their sexual problems from mental health providers. Such help will often be in concert with a physician. In some cases, the collaboration with a physician may merely be that the physician prescribes the medication (such as Viagra in the treatment of erectile dysfunction) while the therapist directs the psychotherapy. In other cases in which the physician may play a more active role, there may be a need for ongoing feedback. For example, in the treatment of vaginismus, there is often a need for the therapist to sensitize the gynecologist to a systematic *in vivo* desensitization strategy to achieve a medical examination. The gynecologist in turn needs to inform the sex therapist of progress in achieving an examination and in the medical results.

The False Dichotomy between Biomedical and Psychosocial Treatment

Some health care providers still dichotomize sexual problems into "organic" and "psychogenic" categories. The assumption is that if the problem has an organic basis, then it has to have an organic solution. This approach does not recognize that many sexual problems emerge from a combination of organic and psychogenic factors; even when the etiology is clearly organic, the best solution may be partly or completely psychological in nature.

As an example of how such a biomedical "fix" can be flawed, consider the following: A woman complains of vaginal dryness and discomfort during sexual intercourse. A purely biomedical approach to treating this problem would probably involve only the prescription of vaginal lubricants. Although such a treatment may be necessary, it may not be sufficient. Perhaps the woman is not sexually aroused because she feels that the relationship, outside as well as inside the bedroom, is unsatisfactory. She would be aroused if her partner expressed affection at other times and were more sensitive to her needs. Because these issues are not addressed by a lubricant, it is likely that the woman will remain unaroused and uncomfortable despite an appropriate (albeit incomplete) treatment.

Similarly, for some men, sexual relations can be dutiful and devoid of satisfying pleasure. The lack of erectile response as a result of diabetes or some other disease process may be met with mixed emotions; that is, a man may feel a loss of masculinity along with the erectile dysfunction. However, this "failure" may provide an acceptable excuse to avoid unsatisfying sexual relations and may be welcomed by both partners. A physician who sees the problem only as a loss of erection may be doing his or her patient a disservice by suggesting a medical solution such as Viagra. The real solution may be to provide the couple with information and to help them overcome restrictive attitudes that have hampered their ability to enjoy coordinated and mutual sensual pleasure in the past.

How to Participate Constructively in Biomedical Approaches to Sexual Health

As a psychosocial consultant to a medical team, you will have an opportunity to affect the system. The extent of your influence will depend upon your ability to work constructively with physicians and to understand the medical approach, as well as your skills as a psychosocial assessor and therapist. Therefore, we devote the remainder of this chapter to discussing how to work with physicians and to help patients use the most common medical interventions.

If you wish to be invited to serve as a consultant, you must gain the respect of physicians by contributing to the care of their patients. Respect may come from the physicians' knowledge of your work and your professional reputation. If you are affiliated with a university or medical school, a certain amount of respect is inherent in your position. If you are not affiliated with a university or medical school, we suggest you build your reputation through contacting and meeting with physicians who are likely to be interested in your services. Regardless of your institutional location, you should make an effort to inform physicians who are most likely to be referral sources (e.g., urologists, gynecologists, family or primary care physicians) that you are interested in treating individuals with sexual problems. If given the opportunity to speak before a group of physicians on the topic of human sexuality, do not decline! This is one of the best opportunities to meet physicians and convey to them your expertise.

Once you have been able to arrange a meeting with a physician, you should convey to him or her that you are interested in being a referral outlet for patients who may require suppplemental psychological/therapeutic intervention. In addition, let the physician know that you may also be called upon to complete a psychosocial evaluation when there is a question of possible psychological or social (i.e., relationship) factors that may be affecting patients' sexual functioning. The physician will find you useful (1) if you can speak to him or her without psychological jargon, (2) if you understand the basic medical aspects of sexual dysfunction, and (3) if you are able to give the physician brief, useful, and timely feedback that will help in his or her treatment.

You will not be perceived as useful if the physician refers a patient but never hears back from you. Your written reports to physicians should contain only the most essential psychosocial history; they should be as brief and to the point as possible. A busy physician has little time for or interest in reading a lengthy report that contains psychological jargon and unsupported inferences regarding family-of-origin conflicts. We suggest that you prepare a succinct, one-page report that identifies the major psychological factors affecting sexual functioning and outlines the treatment plan that you will be recommending (and implementing). As an example, consider Figure 8.1.

How to Help Patients to Use Biomedical Interventions: General Suggestions

The outcome of biomedical assessment of a patient's sexual functioning typically leads to one of three findings: (1) There is clearly no medical condition affecting sexual functioning; (2) there are some signs and symptoms of a med-

---

RE: Mrs. O'Hare

Dear Dr. Richards:

Thank you for referring Mrs. O'Hare to me for evaluation and treatment of her complaint of pain upon intercourse and low sexual desire. I met with Mrs. O'Hare on January 11, 2000, and again on January 27, 2000. I also met separately with Mr. O'Hare on February 1, 2000. Both Mr. and Mrs. O'Hare believe that sexual problems began within the first year of their 12-year marriage and have persisted to the present time.

Mr. and Mrs. O'Hare appear to have a very loving marriage, so I do not feel that the sexual problems are related to marital stress. Rather, it appears that Mrs. O'Hare came from a family background where sexuality was discussed only in negative ways. In addition, she is a person who worries a lot, so she is often distracted (by her worries) even during sex and is unable to focus in a positive way about sex.

Based on your evaluation, which found no medical causes of her sexual problem, and my psychological assessment, I believe that Mrs. O'Hare can benefit from psychotherapy that addresses her negative attitude toward sex and her style of excessive worry. I will continue to see Mrs. O'Hare in therapy and keep you informed.

Thank you for your referral.

Sincerely,

Dr. Prable

FIGURE 8.1. Example of a one-page report.

ical condition that may interfere with sexual functioning; or (3) there is clear-cut evidence that one or more medical conditions are probably interfering with sexual function. Under any of these circumstances, medical intervention may be considered. For example, even when the problem appears to be primarily psychogenic, a noninvasive medical solution (e.g., vacuum device) may be used. At issue is the intensity with which a patient sees the medical intervention as a solution to all of his or her sexual problems. Schover (1989) cautions therapists about patients who insist on a medical solution for their sexual problems. The danger is that in seeking a medical solution, such a patient may be less likely to address important psychosocial issues that may also have an impact on sexual functioning.

In order to help a patient utilize a medical intervention to enhance sexual functioning, the medical intervention must be discussed in the context of a broad view of intimacy and sexuality. Thus, although a woman experiencing painful intercourse may benefit from the use of a lubricant, or a man experiencing erection failure may benefit from vasoactive injections, the use of any medical intervention should be viewed as one component of a therapeutic approach designed to enhance sexual enjoyment. As the therapist, you should be cautious about encouraging a patient to embrace the medical solution if important personal or interpersonal issues remain unresolved. Only when you are confident that your patient can put the medical intervention into perspective should you endorse such an intervention. Schover (1989) has suggested that presence of the following criteria suggest that a patient with an erection problem may not need sex therapy to supplement a biomedical intervention:

1. Good general psychological coping.
2. Good skills on the part of both partners in initiating sex and requesting specific techniques during lovemaking.
3. Agreement between partners on sexual frequency and variety of sexual techniques.
4. Good skills in expressing nonsexual affection.
5. If in a committed relationship, good satisfaction for both partners.
6. History of continuing noncoital sex to orgasm for both partners in spite of an erection problem.
7. If over age 50, good knowledge about sexuality and aging, and how to compensate for minor changes.
8. No sexual dysfunctions other than erectile dysfunction.
9. Clear organic cause for the erectile dysfunction.

Although developed specifically for screening penile prosthesis candidates, we believe that these same criteria are applicable to the treatment of any sexual dysfunction when any medical intervention is being considered. If a patient meets Schover's (1989) criteria, then it is advisable to proceed confidentially with a biomedical intervention. If a patient does not meet all of these criteria, then you should focus on the deficits before recommending the medical intervention. Typically, such therapy focuses on providing information, communication skills, and sexual skills training (see Chapter 7) before proceeding medically.

Suggestions for Specific Biomedical Interventions

In the next section, we describe the types of medical interventions that may be helpful for your patients. Our review focuses disproportionately on male dysfunctions, especially erectile dysfunction; this imbalance reflects the state of the science, that is, relatively little research on biomedical interventions for female sexual dysfunctions, and even less exploring the integration of biomedical and psychosocial approaches (Bartlik & Goldberg, 2000; Binik, Bergeron, & Khalifé, 2000; Heiman, 2000; Leiblum, 2000). We expect this imbalance to begin to reverse during the next decade but, for now, most of the information we provide reflects the greater research base for male dysfunctions.

Pharmacological Approaches

The pharmacological treatments for sexual problems fall into three categories: (1) hormonal therapy (e.g., low testosterone in males treated by injection of testosterone enanthate, or estrogen deficiency in women treated by estrogen replacement therapy); (2) local vasoactive treatments (e.g., erectile dysfunction treated with papaverine, phentolamine, or prostaglandin E1); and (3) oral agents such as Viagra for the treatment of arousal disorders. Of lesser importance is yohimbine (alpha-adrenoreceptor blockers), which is only modestly helpful (Carey & Johnson, 1996), and the medicated urethral system for erection (MUSE; alprostadil), which is the intraurethral suppository form of prostaglandin E1. Delivered by direct insertion into the urethra, MUSE is awkward to use and men tend to prefer Viagra.

HORMONE THERAPY

Low testosterone or elevated prolactin and gonadotropins are hypothesized to cause sexual dysfunction in men. Although the mechanisms by which such hormonal imbalances affect desire or erection remain to be elucidated, testosterone replacement may be suggested by urologists as a treatment for these difficulties. When improvement is seen, it may be due as much to a placebo effect as to a true pharmacological effect. The widespread use of testosterone is most likely influenced by the suspected positive relationship between testosterone and sexual functioning in men, and the small likelihood of side effects. Thus, the philosophy in using testosterone in treating male sexual dysfunction seems to be that it may help to overcome the problem and it cannot hurt. Certainly, there is little evidence that the short-term use of testosterone is harmful, although long-term use in older men may put them at greater risk for hyperplasia (i.e., abnormal growth) of prostate cells (Rous, 1988).

Hormonal problems that affect sexual functioning in women most commonly occur during menopause or postmenopause. (They can also occur prematurely as a result of surgical treatment for cancer.) Women experiencing lowered levels of estrogen may be susceptible to shrinking and thinning of the vagina, a loss of tissue elasticity, and lessened vaginal lubrication during sexual arousal (Masters, Johnson, & Kolodny, 1988). The decrease in vaginal lubrication often results in dyspareunia if an artificial lubricant is not used. Research investigating the effects of hormone replacement therapy (HRT) on sexual outcomes has been reviewed by Walling, Andersen, and Johnson (1990). These authors concluded that estrogen therapy leads to significant gynecological improvements (e.g., reduced atrophic vaginitis) which may, in turn, allow sexual functioning to return to normal. Progestogen therapy, on the other hand, provides few, if any, direct sexual benefits, but it is useful because it reduces the risk of endometrial hyperplasia, which can occur with estrogen therapy alone.

Hormonal therapy has been also used to treatment sexual dysfunction in postmenopausal women. Sarrel (2000) reviewed the literature and concluded that dyspareunia due to vaginal dryness appears to be most responsive to estrogen replacement therapy (ERT); however, progestins can oppose these changes and lead to a recurrence of dryness and dyspareunia. ERT has also been reported to enhance sexual desire in some women. According to Sarrel, treatment with ERT can be helpful for many women, but there are others whose sexual difficulties remain unresponsive. There also appears to be a significant subgroup of women whose sexual difficulties respond initially to ERT but who subsequently revert to their initial problems, especially when the problem is low desire. For these women, the addition of androgen may be helpful.

Much remains to be known about which women are likely to require (and respond to) HRT as well as what type, dose, duration, and route of administration will prove optimal. Although no major breakthroughs have been realized in the last 10 years pertaining to the pharmacological treatment of female sexual dysfunction (Heiman & Meston, 1997), many investigators are optimistic about the next decade of research (Bartlik & Goldberg, 2000).

VASOACTIVE THERAPY

Vasoactive injection of phenoxybenzamine was first reported by Brindley (1983) to induce successful erections. Since Brindley's early report, other agents [i.e., papavarine hydrochloride, phentolamine mesylate, and prosta-glandin E1 (PGE-1)] have all been shown to effectively increase erectile re-sponse (Linet & Neff, 1994; Mahmoud, El Dakhil, Fahjmi & Abdel-Aziz, 1992). Vasoactive injection therapy, although effective, has a high dropout rate (Turner & Althof, 1992). Additionally, once Viagra became available, men strongly preferred taking a pill to injecting themselves in the penis. Nonethe-less, for a limited number of men, Viagra does not work but vasoactive injec-tions do. We continue to be cautious about any medical procedure that focuses solely on function rather than on the enhancement of the broader intimate rela-tionship between two people. For those selected cases in which vasoactive in-jections are indicated, sex therapy can help sustain the long-term beneficial use and reduce unwanted psychological side effects such as partner dissatis-faction and low arousal.

VIAGRA (SILDENAFIL CITRATE)

Since its release in 1998, Viagra has revolutionized the treatment of erectile dysfunction. All other treatments for erectile disorder experienced almost an immediate decline in use, including vasoactive injections, vacuum devices, MUSE, and implant surgery. However, as time has passed, there has been a re-bound in all of these other treatments because Viagra is not effective for every-one. Current use has certainly not reached the pre-Viagra levels, but there have been increases, nonetheless, and these other procedures are still viable.

Viagra works through a chain of biochemical events that results in smooth muscle relaxation and inflow of blood to the corpus cavernosum. This occurs only during sexual stimulation. Taking Viagra in the absence of sexual stimulation will not normally result in an erection, although we have had some men report spontaneous erections without direct stimulation following Viagra ingestion. We have also had a number of men report firmer morning erections even though the Viagra was taken the previous night. Viagra is supposed to have an effective half-life of 4–6 hours.

Working in conjunction with a physician, we find Viagra to be a useful adjunct to a psychosocial approach for treating erectile disorder. Many of our patients have reported increases in their sexual confidence level once they know that Viagra works. We advise patients to try Viagra during masturbation (only if this is a comfortable practice) to get used to it and to determine if there are any side effects. Viagra is not recommended for men with a heart condition who are taking nitrate-based medications, nor for men with retinitis pigmentosa. Assuming there are no contraindications, a small percentage of men taking Viagra report headaches (16%) and flushing (10%).

Men with no organic basis for erectile disorder often find that once Viagra works for them, they do not need to use it every time. In fact, these men have repeatedly told us that just knowing that they have Viagra as a "back up" gives them the confidence to engage in sexual relationships again.

At this time, there are no large-scale controlled research studies with women to support the efficacy of Viagra for treating sexual dysfunction. Small-sample studies have demonstrated mixed results. The next few years should bring us evidence regarding the efficacy of Viagra and other pharmacological agents for the treatment of female sexual dysfunction.

Surgery

Surgical treatment of the female sexual dysfunctions continues to be relatively infrequent, but several recent studies have evaluated the surgical treatment of severe vulvar vestibulitis. Bergeron, Bouchard, Fortier, Binik, and Khalifé (1997) evaluated the long-term (3 years) effectiveness of vestibulectomy in relieving coital pain and improving sexual function in 38 women. Surgery yielded a positive outcome for two-thirds of the women and moderate to no improvement for the other one-third. McCormack and Spence (1999) followed 42 women who had undergone surgery for approximately 5 years. They found that 28 (85%) of 33 sexually active women who had dyspareunia before surgery reported that intercourse was much less painful or pain-free following surgery. Bornstein, Goldik, Stolar, Zarfati, and Abramovici (1997) sought to predict the outcome of surgery in a sample of 79 women. They compared women who experienced a complete response (76%) to those (24%) who had an incomplete response. These two groups were similar in all comparisons except for constant vulvar pain of vestibular origin (in addition to dyspareunia) and the presence of symptoms since first coitus. They concluded that an incomplete response to surgery may be anticipated in women with vulvar vestibulitis associated with dyspareunia since their first episode of intercourse and in those with associated vulvar pain. Treatment approaches other than surgery should be considered for such patients. We look forward to increased multidisciplinary research in the next decade to tell us more about the psychosocial aspects of these procedures, as well as studies regarding appropriate candidates for surgical interventions.

There are three surgical approaches to treating male erectile problems: (1) the implantable penile prosthesis, (2) penile arterial revascularization, and (3) penile venous ligation. As in the case of pharmacological approaches to sexual dysfunctions, there is a gap in the literature regarding the psychological concomitants of surgical intervention (Mendoza & Silverman, 1987). The surgical perspective has focused almost entirely on improvement in surgical procedures to produce a firmer and more natural erection with the fewest medical complications. In evaluating the effectiveness of surgical procedures, infection rates, mechanical malfunction, and medical complications are reported. When patient satisfaction is included in the evaluation process, it is almost always presented in global terms of "satisfied" or "not satisfied." Schover (1989) points out that such an approach to assessment is flawed because of the principle of cognitive dissonance (i.e., the more effort that a man expends, and the more difficulty he endures in order to reach the goal, the more he may be expected to value that attainment, regardless of the "objective" outcome). Thus, men who go through the pain and expense of surgery will be likely to take a positive view of their postoperative functioning.

PENILE PROSTHESES

Surgical procedures to improve male sexual functioning have existed since the beginning of the 20th century. Credit for the development of the modern penile prosthesis is given to Small, Carrion, and Gordon (1975) for the semirigid silicone prosthesis, and to Scott, Bradley, and Timm (1973) for the inflatable prosthesis. These devices were considerable improvements over the earlier devices, which utilized rib cartilage, were prone to ulceration, and lacked malleability. The use of the semirigid silicone rod or the inflatable prosthesis provides a close semblance to normal functioning, with an acceptable level of side effects.

Since the late 1980s, the importance of psychosocial factors in implant surgery has been addressed (e.g., Krauss, Lantinga, Carey, Meisler, & Kelly, 1989; Meisler, Carey, Krauss, & Lantinga, 1988; Pedersen, Teifer, Ruiz, & Melman, 1988; Schover, 1989; Tiefer, Pedersen, & Melman, 1988). Research has sought to identify psychosocial predictors of positive outcomes. As mentioned earlier, Schover (1989) has outlined factors associated with positive outcome following penile implant. Meisler et al. (1988) offer additional support for Schover's (1989) observation; they describe a case in which poor psychological coping and poor marital adjustment prior to the implant was associated with a negative postsurgical adjustment.

The collaborative relationship between sex therapists and urologists is extremely important in the screening of potential implant patients. Some urologists may look upon psychologists only in terms of a resource for screening out poor candidates and treating psychopathology. However, as Schover's (1989) work suggests, even in cases with a clear organic basis, there is a need to attend to subtle factors related to overall sexual and relationship skills. Furthermore, it is important to assess a patient's sexual expectations, attitudes, and knowledge. For example, if a man is single and has avoided all social and sexual contact (because he believes that a firm erection is essential for a relationship with any woman), then that man is a poor candidate for surgery. Such a man is likely to have complaints and insecurities about the size and firmness of his "implanted" penis; he is also likely to engage in sexual activity to "prove" masculinity rather than because he is involved in a close and loving relationship with a partner. The desire to prove one's masculinity through sexual expression often results in other (e.g., orgasmic) problems.

As a sex therapist, you can assist in the assessment and treatment of potential implant patients because of your skills in interviewing and psychological assessment; moreover, you can take the time that most surgeons do not have to extract the subtle information necessary for accurate screening. In some cases, it is only necessary to ask more detailed questions to arrive at an accurate presurgical decision.

Although implant surgery is still performed as a viable treatment of erectile disorder, there are certainly fewer candidates now than there were in the 1980s. Less invasive, effective treatments for erectile disorder now exist that were not available in the 1980s. Men who would have been considered previously for a penile implant are now being treated with less invasive procedures, such as Viagra.

VASCULAR SURGERY

As discussed in Chapter 3, there are two categories of vascular problems that may affect erectile functioning: arterial (i.e., inflow) decrease and/or venous (i.e., outflow) increase. Arterial problems result when there is a narrowing or blockage of the pudendal or dorsal penile arteries that supply blood to the corpora cavernosa. The engorgement of blood in the corpora cavernosa is necessary for the erection to occur. In order for the erection to be maintained, blood has to be "trapped" in the corpora cavernosa at a certain pressure. If too much blood circulates out of the penis or "leaks," the erection will subside. This is a problem of venous leakage.

Surgical procedures to correct both arterial and venous problems have been employed since the early part of this century, with somewhat uncertain results (Hawatmeh, Houttuin, Gregory, & Purcell, 1983). Advances in the understanding of the physiology of the erectile response have led to improved surgical procedures with some claims of success (Balko et al., 1986; Bennett, 1988; Lewis, 1988). However, long-term follow-up studies are lacking in this area; although the immediate results of vascular surgery are often successful, follow-up evaluation 6–9 months after surgery often reports high failure rates. Lewis (1988) reviewed the literature on venous surgery and concluded that failure occurs in about 50% of the cases. Rossman, Mieza, and Melman (1990) have reported a failure rate of about 90% with venous surgery at 9 months postsurgery. They conclude that there may be a defect in the active veno-occlusive mechanism in these patients that the surgery does not correct.

An exception to these results was provided by Kayigil, Ahmed, and

Metin (2000), who reported on their experiences with one type of vascular surgery, deep dorsal vein arterialization, in a specialized series of 25 younger men. With a mean follow-up of 28 months, about three-fourths of the men were judged successful at a 1-year follow-up, and two-thirds at 2- and 3-year follow-up. However, the younger age of their sample may have made interpreting their results somewhat difficult.

The psychological consideration for vascular surgery candidates should be similar to that for implant surgery candidates. A cost–benefit analysis should be made, and presurgical therapy should be considered for patients who do not demonstrate the positive predictors outlined by Schover (1989). Patients who have avoided all sexual interactions for several months or more, or patients who show evidence of marital difficulties, could benefit from presurgical therapy.

An important difference exists between vascular surgery and either implant or vasoactive injection, namely, if the vascular surgery is successful, then "natural" functioning is restored. Thus, men who undergo successful vascular surgery will obtain erections only when (1) there is sufficient erotic stimulation, and (2) they desire sex. On the other hand, men with implants or vasoactive injections may participate in sex without sufficient erotic stimulation or feelings of desire. Sex under such conditions, as discussed earlier, may be highly unsatisfactory and iatrogenic for the man and his partner.

Vacuum Device Therapy

The use of vacuum devices for assisting men to obtain erections has been sanctioned by the medical profession since the 1980s (Nadig, Ware, & Blumoff, 1986). Several devices are currently being marketed; most work by creating a vacuum in a cylinder, which is placed over the penis. The vacuum draws blood into the corpora cavernosa of the penis; this blood is then trapped by placing a constricting "rubber band" around the base of the penis.

Although such a procedure "works" (i.e., produces an erection) for most men (even those whose erectile difficulties are organically based), it is not without problems. First, it takes some dexterity to manipulate the pumping device in the manner needed to complete a seal around the base of the penis. Second, once the desired degree of tumescence is reached (some men report pain in the penis during the pumping process), the constricting band must be slipped off the cylinder and onto the base of the penis; in this process, the band itself may cause some discomfort. Third, ecchymosis (i.e., bruises) and petachiae (i.e., red spots) are reported in some men, although these are reversed with a period of disuse.

Nadig et al. (1986) note that the erection created by the vacuum device differs from a naturally occurring erection in five ways. First, the blood flow into the penis decreases while the rubber bands are in place. Second, penile skin temperature falls as a result of decreased arterial blood flow. Third, the penile circumference increases more with this device than during normal erections. Fourth, the penis is rigid only distal to the constrictive bands and thus pivots at its base. And, finally, the ejaculate is trapped in the proximal urethra until the bands are removed; thus, men using the device do not ejaculate as they have previously, even though they do experience an orgasm.

In spite of these differences, some short-term follow-up studies have reported about 80% satisfaction with the vacuum devices (Nadig et al., 1986; Viosca & Griner, 1988; Witherington, 1988). However, the device is clearly not for everyone. For example, Earle et al. (1996) surveyed 60 men who tried the vacuum erection device; only 43 of the 60 men responded to the survey and, of these, most (81%) reported that they had abandoned the device. The primary reason given was that "it did not work." Delizonna et al. (2001) reported that the production of an erection solely through the use of a vacuum device did not evoke subjective feelings of sexual arousal. This study lends support to the crucial importance of the sexual environment whenever a purely medical approach is utilized.

In one of the few studies with a long-term follow-up, Derouet, Caspari, Rohde, Rommel, and Ziegler (1999) followed 190 patients. Of these, only 110 patients (58%) answered the questionnaire; 20% of these men rejected the device immediately and another 31% rejected it after a period of up to 16 weeks. Only 42% were long-term users (with a median use time of 28 months). Long-term users—mainly patients who did not respond to other treatments—and their partners tended to be satisfied with the vacuum therapy and complications were minor. Based on these studies, it seems that few men like the vacuum device; however, for these men, vacuum therapy appears to be a safe and effective, noninvasive treatment. There remains a need for more long-term studies (i.e., lasting a year or more) that evaluate the impact of such a device on the sexual satisfaction of the patient and his partner, and to determine who likes the devise.

We would advise that men who are considering vacuum devices go through the same psychological screening as that of implant candidates. It is important that the man and his partner have realistic expectations for the use of the device and not expect it to solve relationship problems. All of the considerations for implant therapy candidates raised by Schover (1989) apply to the vacuum device candidate. A final point about the vacuum device: It may also be used as a diagnostic tool for implant candidates about whom there is some doubt. Because the vacuum device is noninvasive, there are fewer problems that may occur if the device does not work. If a man and his partner have difficulty with, or complaints about, the use of the vacuum device, it is likely that they would also have difficulty with the implant.

Concluding Comments

The complexity of sexual problems for both men and women demands the most comprehensive treatment approach possible. Poor success rates, high attrition rates and patient dissatisfaction are common to both purely psychosocial (Baggaley, Hirst, & Watson, 1996) and biomedical treatments (Kim & Lipshultz, 1997; Pedersen & Mohl, 1991; Sundaram et al., 1997). There is an increasing recognition that combination treatments are necessary (Heiman & Meston, 1997). With this recognition, there is a greater need for cooperation between biomedical and psychosocial providers. Several recent multi-disciplinary conferences provide evidence that this cooperation is under way (Goldstein, 1999; O'Leary & Rosen, 1997, 1998).

9

Case Illustrations

The seven cases presented in this chapter were seen by us and were selected to illustrate a range of commonly encountered clinical situations. All cases include pertinent diagnostic information but identifying information has been changed to protect patient confidentiality.

Case 1: Ms. Jones (Orgasmic Disorder)

Ms. Jones, a 40-year-old divorced mother of two, presented with a complaint of orgasmic disorder. She had been divorced for 4 years following a bitter, 10-year marriage. She had experienced orgasm with other partners during college but not during her marriage nor subsequently with new partners. Ms. Jones presented with a great deal of anxiety, self-blame, and emotional lability over this problem. Similar to men experiencing erectile disorder, Ms. Jones expressed performance fears and interpreted her lack of orgasm as a statement of her gender inadequacy: Because she could not reach orgasm, she did not feel like a woman.

Assessment

During the intake interview, Ms. Jones revealed that she had not had a gynecological examination for several years. She acknowledged that she had avoided an examination because of her fear that a medical doctor might not take her complaint seriously. After discussion, she agreed that a medical examination was important and made arrangements with a female gynecologist known to handle sexual concerns in a sensitive manner.

In the medical examination, all indications were that Ms. Jones was healthy, and that there were no medical explanations for her lack of orgasm.

Ms. Jones revealed that she was left alone a lot by her parents and, as a result, had always feared abandonment. Both parents also blamed her a lot and rarely praised her. She felt that she stayed in her failed marriage, even though she knew it was wrong from the start, mainly because she felt she was to blame for the marital problems (her husband told her so). She also feared being left alone. Although she finally gathered the courage to leave what had become a verbally abusive marriage, she carried with her the guilt about its failure. Her lack of orgasm was cited by her husband as a sign of her inadequacy and a source of his dissatisfaction. She had fully accepted the premise that her sexual problem had caused the breakup of the marriage rather than entertaining the idea that lack of a rewarding relationship from the start contributed to her sexual unresponsiveness.

She would "try" very hard to achieve orgasm through masturbation and despite becoming increasingly frustrated would persist as long as 30 minutes or more. At times, she would stop because she was actually irritating herself and causing pain. After she entered therapy, she had decided not to date at all because she felt inadequate.

Case Formulation and Treatment Plan

Ms. Jones suffered from acquired, generalized, female orgasmic disorder because of her history of being capable of orgasm when circumstances were favorable. However, because of her family background, she readily accepted blame, misattributing her lack of sexual arousal and orgasm to her own shortcomings rather than to marital incompatibility (or other external factors). Her husband, in a manner similar to her mother, blamed her for almost all problems, including sex. Convinced of her sexual inadequacy, she worried about her sexual performance beyond the marriage, into subsequent relationships and masturbation. In all respects, she manifested classic performance anxiety. The treatment plan was to address first the self-blame and misattributions regarding the cause of her sexual difficulties, and only then to move on to a sensate focus approach. If the self-blame and misattributions were not addressed first, we hypothesized that the sensate focus treatment alone would fail.

Treatment

Therapy began with teaching Ms. Jones about the importance of positive attitudes, relationships, and environment in order to achieve a satisfying sexual relationship. We emphasized the importance of a positive, loving partnership and also explained that regardless of the original cause of her sexual difficulties, her focus on performance was interfering with positive erotic thoughts that would facilitate desire, arousal, and orgasm.

Once Ms. Jones was able to understand and accept the notion that, like everyone else, she needed to consider the importance of sexually positive circumstances, she was able to stop blaming herself and to proceed more positively. She agreed that she had focused entirely on producing an orgasm and not at all on her mood or the presence of erotic stimulation. In therapy, we instructed her to masturbate but not achieve orgasm and to pay attention to mood, erotic feelings/fantasies, and sensations. Masturbation was to last no more than 15 minutes and Ms. Jones was to stop if she felt herself getting close to orgasm.

The masturbatory sensate focus approach worked extremely well and Ms. Jones was able to shift her focus to creating the right environment for sex (positive mood, relaxed time, privacy, erotic thoughts). Additionally, she was able to identify increasing arousal and unexpectedly achieved orgasm. After discussion about selecting a partner who was not only attractive to her but also understanding, and who did not place demands on her or pressure her for sex we then encouraged her to date. This case involved a total of 11 sessions over 6 months.

Case 2: Mr. And Mrs. Law (Male Low Arousal and Sexual Disinterest)

Mr. and Mrs. Law, both in their early 40s and college educated, had been married for 12 years with 2 children. The presenting complaint was that Mr. Law was not interested in sex with Mrs. Law. She felt angry, rejected, and was considering separation. Mr. Law said he was interested in sex with his wife but his busy profession left him tired and without desire, energy, or time.

Assessment

We conducted separate initial interviews, following the typical protocol. The interview with Mrs. Law revealed that she came from a wealthy family but always felt overshadowed by her more attractive, older sister. Her parents were insensitive to this issue and, in fact, were very critical of her. Her self-esteem was further damaged by many rejections from boys during her teenage years. Although she blossomed in college, she continued to have a poor self-image. She stated that she loved her husband but felt rejected by him.

Mr. Law came from a lower-middle-class family and was raised by a somewhat distant father and an emotionally labile, alcoholic mother. He recalled his father silently taking verbal abuse from his mother and then exploding in anger. Mr. Law had forged a very successful professional career and did feel very pressured in trying to balance career and family. He described his wife as very angry much of the time and felt like he was walking on eggshells. He expressed love for his wife and said that he did not want to separate or divorce.

An exchange that characterized the couple's communication was relayed as follows: Mrs. Law found a letter to Mr. Law from a female whom she did not know. She immediately concluded that her husband was having an affair with this woman, since their own sex life was so poor. Because they had not had sex in several months, in her mind, the only logical explanation was an affair, and the only logical solution was divorce. Upon arriving home from work, Mr. Law was confronted angrily by his wife. She would not tell him about the letter, only that she had evidence of his affair and wanted a divorce. He responded to her anger by calling her crazy and withdrawing. She persisted until he exploded and walked out of the house. (Incidentally, the letter was a thank-you note from a former secretary, an elderly woman for whom he had done some favors.)

Case Formulation and Treatment Plan

The assessment revealed that Mr. Law had acquired, specific, hypoactive sexual desire disorder. His low desire was specific to his wife but not to other women. When the couple was getting along, Mr. Law did feel some sexual desire for his wife. Because of the specificity of the problem to his wife, we focused treatment on trying to improve positive feelings and communication between them, helping Mrs. Law with anger control, and Mr. Law with being more sensitive to his wife's needs.

Treatment

Due to the level of anger and the obvious presence of cognitive distortions and faulty communication styles, we began therapy with communication training. In addition, we implemented a date night (with each partner alternately responsible for the planning) and set up specific times during the week to practice communication. We explained that this first phase of therapy was necessary before directly addressing the sexual issues. We also explained and they understood (on an intellectual level) that there was no evidence of low sexual desire; rather, the sexual avoidance was a result of anger. Conflicts were so frequent and so explosive that positive feelings and trust were mostly absent.

Initially, the couple worked diligently on improving communication and correcting cognitive distortions, and, as we predicted, sexual activity increased as positive feelings returned. However, in spite of relapse prevention training, Mrs. Law would occasionally lapse into old patterns. Her insecurities would get the best of her and she would explode with jealousy and make extreme and caustic remarks. These episodes, although less frequent than before, were no less damaging and resulted in clear setbacks whenever they occurred. Mr. and Mrs. Law demonstrated some positive changes but were still encountering difficulties after a year of therapy. They agreed to stay together and continue to work on their relationship, but they dropped out of therapy after 18 sessions.

Case 3: Mr. Konrad (Erectile Disorder)

Mr. Konrad, a 50-year-old, single, gay male, who worked as an executive in a medium-size company, had broken up with his longtime partner about a year before seeking therapy. He was experiencing erectile dysfunction with new partners. He stated that he had met a new, younger partner (age 39) with whom he was hoping to establish a long-term relationship. Mr. Konrad was unable to obtain an erection in three sexual encounters and was very concerned about losing this new partner because of his erection difficulties.

Assessment

Mr. Konrad described his parents as withholding warmth and affection, and undermining his self-esteem. He had always struggled with self-esteem issues in spite of rather impressive achievements in school and at work. A full medical examination, including a hormonal assessment, revealed no medical explanation for his erectile dysfunction. He reported achieving full NPT response but was worried because he did not wake up with a full erection every morning.

He acknowledged that he had placed his new partner on a pedestal and that he was focused on performing sexually out of a fear that this younger partner would reject him. He had absolutely no problem in maintaining a full erection during masturbation but failed with his partner in spite of his partner's reassurance.

Mr. Konrad stated that he was comfortable with his homosexuality and had been "out" since his teenage years. Although his goal was to settle down into a long-term monogamous relationship that did not focus on sex, he felt that he had to live up to the very strong emphasis on sexual performance in the "gay world."

Case Formulation and Treatment Plan

The assessment revealed that Mr. Konrad suffered from acquired specific male erectile disorder. All assessment information pointed to misinformation and performance anxiety as the likely causes of Mr. Konrad's erectile dysfunction. He accepted this explanation but also wanted to explore the possibility of

Viagra as a treatment option. Thus, the treatment plan was to focus initially on providing accurate information to clear up misunderstandings, use sensate focus to address performance anxiety, and prescribe Viagra as a backup "safety net" to supplement the sex therapy.

Treatment

Treatment involved correcting some sexual myths that Mr. Konrad endorsed; for example, we informed him that his view that men should awaken with a firm erection every morning was not accurate. Also, we encouraged Mr. Konrad to try a (nondemand) sensate focus exercise with his partner before using Viagra. His partner was very cooperative and, indeed, this plan worked very well. Mr. Konrad felt very relaxed and for the first time achieved a full erection with his partner.

Even though he was pleased with his erection and more confident in his sexual ability, Mr. Konrad wished to also explore the use of Viagra "as a backup." We discussed the pros and cons of this strategy thoroughly and Mr. Konrad chose to try out the Viagra. Consistent with therapeutic instructions, he first took Viagra to determine if there were any side effects (starting with 50 mg). He initially planned to test it out during masturbation. To his surprise, he experienced a full erection soon after his initial dose, while walking around his home. His plan was to attempt masturbation about an hour after ingestion but, according to him, the rubbing of his pants was enough to stimulate an erection.

In a follow-up session 2 months later, Mr. Konrad reported that his sex life was completely back to normal and he had only used Viagra once. He stated that just knowing the Viagra was there had been very reassuring to him even if he never used it again. This is an example of the positive use of Viagra in combination with the usual psychotherapeutic approach for erectile disorder. Sensate focus strategy, along with a relapse prevention approach, helped to focus Mr. Konrad's sexual interests and avoid pitfalls of negative sexual thoughts and experiences. The Viagra helped as an additional reassurance and confidence booster. The treatment and follow-up took a total of 10 sessions over 6 months.

Case 4: Mr. and Mrs. Dennison
(Vaginismus)

Mr. and Mrs. Dennison were in their mid-20s and married 1 year when they first came to therapy. Mrs. Dennison felt very uncomfortable about sexual relations. The couple had been unable to complete intercourse even though they had tried numerous times. On each occasion, Mrs. Dennison had tensed up, cried, and felt pain in her vagina. The couple were very loving toward one another and expressed strong physical attraction. In addition, they communicated very openly, without blaming one another about the problem. Mr. Dennison was patient, did not place demands on Mrs. Dennison, and was sensitive to her problem.

Assessment

As recommended in Chapter 6, Mr. And Mrs. Dennison were interviewed separately. She was one of four children and came from a very religious background. Both of her parents were alcoholics but showed affection both toward her and each other. As a teenager, Mrs. Dennison had severe acne and never dated any boys. Her mother consistently warned her not to get pregnant. Furthermore, nudity in front of others was not allowed in the home and Mrs. Dennison always felt uncomfortable looking at her body in a mirror; she also felt uncomfortable in all but a very conservative one-piece bathing suit.

Although Mrs. Dennison could insert tampons and tolerate a gynecological examination, she was unable to look at or touch her vagina when she was naked. She did not allow Mr. Dennison to touch her vagina, and she did not want Mr. Dennison to see her naked. She also reported that she did not want to touch her husband's penis and expressed great disgust regarding the thought of sperm on her body and oral sex. She seemed to have a very low tolerance for pain and noted that her body was unusually sensitive. She also felt that her vagina might be anatomically different from that of other women and more at an angle that promoted pain. Her gynecologist reassured her that she was anatomically and medically normal.

Mr. Dennison, on the other hand, was very comfortable sexually in spite of only limited experience with one other partner. Both his parents were very loving and he was confident, with very adequate self-esteem.

Case Formulation and Treatment Plan

The assessment revealed that Iris suffered from lifelong, specific vaginismus. The specificity was to sexual but not nonsexual situations. Negative sexual messages, religiosity, and poor self-image all contributed to the problem. Because the couple communicated well and had a positive relationship, the treatment plan focused on challenging Iris's automatic, negative sex messages and desensitizing her to sexual fears.

Treatment

Although there were numerous barriers to sexual intercourse and many other aspects of sexual relations, there were some encouraging signs. Mr. and Mrs. Dennison were very attracted to and loving toward each other. They enjoyed kissing and breast stimulation. Surprisingly, Iris also could masturbate to orgasm by stimulating herself through her clothing. Her ability to do this provided her with the understanding that sex could be pleasurable. Women without this experience have much more difficulty in accepting the concept that sex can be pleasurable.

Treatment was structured to include both individual strategies for Mrs. Dennison and couple strategies. We encouraged her in individual efforts to begin by saying sexual words and looking at herself nude in the mirror. This *in vivo* desensitization was accompanied by cognitive restructuring. Her automatic negative thoughts generally undermined her self-confidence and contaminated her sexual experience; we needed to challenge and reframe these thoughts.

The couple was also instructed in an *in vivo* desensitization procedure that began with the partners lying next to each other fully clothed and embracing. As in the individual practice sessions, Mrs. Dennison was instructed to challenge any automatic negative thoughts that emerged during couple practice.

The couple was also given instructions as follows: If Mr. Dennison became aroused and he or Mrs. Dennison was comfortable, then stimulation to orgasm/ejaculation was permissible. A hierarchy of sexual behaviors was identified and the couple focused on the specific components of the hierarchy in a step-by-step fashion. To help desensitize her to sperm, she was instructed to practice holding white liquid soap in her hand and placing it on her body. This greatly assisted the process, and when Mr. Dennison finally did ejaculate during a sensate focus session, she was able to touch the sperm with only mild disturbance. Eventually, she was able to lie comfortably for up to 20 minutes, with sperm on her body before washing.

A serendipitous experience helped contribute to further improvement. On one occasion, while at a friend's wedding, Mrs. Dennison had a couple of glasses of wine. Apparently, the wine and the joy of the occasion inspired her to lead Mr. Dennison into a spare room at the country club and attempt sexual relations. She later reported that she had never experienced such sexual desire, and had it not been for the intrusive knocking at the door by the flower girl, she was convinced that she would have enjoyed penetration.

This experience helped the couple to move forward in their sensate focus practice to begin practicing penile–vaginal insertion. Without wine and song, the practice took longer than expected, but, eventually, penetration was achieved. As in the individual practice sessions, Mrs. Dennison was instructed to challenge any automatic negative thoughts that emerged during couple practice. In spite of all of the positive ingredients present for this couple (love, attraction, intelligence, excellent communication), the therapy process was lengthy. Avoidance and erratic practice contributed to delays. It was not the lack of motivation but rather the strength of the anxiety and entrenchment of the negative thinking that delayed the process.

In the end, the couple was able to enjoy intercourse without pain, although Mrs. Dennison did not become comfortable inserting her own finger in her vagina. Mr. Dennison could insert his finger, but she could not insert her own finger even though she knew this was irrational. She learned to manipulate her husband's penis very comfortably and could experience ejaculate on her body without becoming distressed. Although ultimately successful, this case typifies the emotionality often involved in overcoming vaginismus and points to the need to address cognitive factors along with an *in vivo* desensitization approach. Therapy took a total of 25 sessions over a 2-year period.

Case 5: Ms. Simon (Low Desire)

Ms. Simon, a 35-year-old divorcée who presented with low sexual desire, was involved in a relationship with a man and reported that she was avoiding sex because of low sexual desire, and that all of her relationships with men, including a 6-year marriage, started with high sexual interest and then evolved to low sexual interest and even sexual aversion. It was very confusing to her (and to her partners) that she could be initially very sexually assertive and adventurous but then become sexually avoidant.

Assessment

Ms. Simon presented a very complex and interesting history that elucidated her seemingly paradoxical behavior. She was raised as the youngest child in a family of five children. Her parents were very religious and sexually repressive; they also made her feel unattractive and inferior to others. There was never any nudity in the home; the word "sex" was never uttered. She remembered not being allowed to see her high school play, *West Side Story*, because her parents objected to the "sex" in the play.

In spite of her feelings of inferiority and unattractiveness, she was in reality an attractive, bright woman. In high school, she was surprised when boys were attracted to her. She complied with any sexual advances in a new relationship in order to keep her partner interested. The cycle of sexual interest and disinterest seemed to be best explained as a result of inferiority feelings that led to desperation and sexual compliance in the initial stage of a relationship and, later, to feelings of being used, followed by her rejection of her partners. Furthermore, we learned that she, not surprisingly, had very negative feelings toward sex. Her sexual involvement with a new partner was labeled by her as positive because of her desperation to make the relationship work. The novelty of a new relationship apparently overrode her deeply felt negative feelings about sex.

Case Formulation and Treatment Plan

This case is an example of lifelong, specific, hypoactive sexual desire disorder. The assessment and formulation identified several important issues that had to be addressed in treatment. First, sexual misinformation and automatic negative thinking had to be addressed. She was unassertive, felt inferior, and had many negative thoughts. Helping her understand the relationship between her upbringing, and her negative sexual image and negative sexual thoughts, was the starting point of treatment, which included a combination of sexual information, cognitive restructuring, assertiveness training, and *in vivo* desensitization.

Treatment

Once Ms. Simon understood the relationship between her upbringing and her negative self-image and maladaptive sexual attitudes, she was able to move forward and stop blaming herself. She responded well to cognitive restructuring of negative self-statements and practiced accepting, rather than negating, compliments of friends. She also benefited from writing a list of her positive attributes and accomplishments. Sexually, she practiced desensitizing herself to viewing her naked body in the mirror and looking at sexual activity of couples depicted in *The New Joy of Sex and More Joy of Sex* (Comfort, 1998). Finally, she practiced being more assertive with a new boyfriend and was able to limit sexual activity to what she wanted and not always give in to what her new partner wanted.

Therapy involved 16 sessions over a 6-month period. At the end of therapy, Ms. Simon felt more positive about herself and enjoyed sexual activity.

Case 6: Mr. Gordon (Low Desire)

Mr. Gordon, a 55-year-old, divorced, health care professional, presented with a complaint of low sexual desire. He had been dating a 45-year-old woman for the past year and expressed great fondness for her. In spite of having a very warm and loving relationship with his new partner, Mr. Gordon expressed concern over his lack of sexual desire. He had not attempted sexual relations with her. In the past, he had at times experienced strong sexual desire and satisfactory sexual relations with women, and he had also experienced sexual desire for men.

Assessment

During the assessment, he disclosed that he had always been strongly attracted to men. He rejected acting on these attractions and preferred to pursue heterosexual relations. Throughout his life, he had a number of heterosexual relations, including his 10-year marriage. Because he has also experienced intense arousal with men and women, he considered himself to be a bisexual.

He recalled that, at age 11, he and a male friend used to lie in bed together and fondle each other's penises while looking at *Playboy* magazines. Additionally, he recalled being fondled during the same time period by a neighborhood man. As a teen, he had "crushes" on males but dated females; however, he avoided sex with females.

It also appeared that, in early childhood, he may have developed some negative attitudes and feelings toward sex with females due to his mother's inappropriate warnings about sex. His mother repeatedly told him that she would cut his penis off if he ever had sex with a girl. He heeded his mother's threats and, not surprisingly, avoided all sexual contacts with females as a teen. He did, however, date females and had his first sexual intercourse experience with a girl in college. He stated that he enjoyed his initial sexual experience. Thus, what evolved for Mr. Gordon was a history of strong sexual attraction for males (which he never acted on) and mild sexual attractions for females (which he successfully acted on and enjoyed).

He married a college girlfriend and had two sons. He stayed married for 10 years and remained faithful to his wife but found that he became less interested in sex, which he believes contributed to the dissolution of his marriage.

Following his divorce, he dated several different women and had a very intense and enjoyable sexual relationship with one woman for a 6-month period. Each of these relationships ended, however, for a variety of reasons. He very deliberately chose not to act on his homosexual attractions. His executive role in a large company was highly visible, and he did not want to jeopardize his position by engaging in relationships with men, and possibly being discovered.

In his most current relationship, he found a partner who shared many of his values and interests. He very much wanted the relationship to be successful but he was cautious about a long-term commitment. He was receiving pressure from his partner to consider marriage.

Case Formulation and Treatment Plan

This case demonstrates lifelong, specific, hypoactive sexual desire disorder. Although Mr. Gordon experienced less desire for his current girlfriend than he had for some previous female partners, and less desire than what he experienced toward males during masturbation fantasies, it seemed that he was avoiding sex because of fear of commitment. His low desire was specific to females in a committed relationship. The treatment plan focused on (a) increasing his comfort with sexual orientation and lifestyle issues, and (b) clarifying the type of relationship he wished to establish with his girlfriend.

Treatment

Therapy helped Mr. Gordon to better define and delineate his sexual identity, orientation, and interests. Although he had recognized his bisexuality, he had not clearly understood possible factors that contributed to his sexual development. Furthermore, he had not understood various factors that influenced or interfered with the fluctuations in the strength of his sexual desire (i.e., fear of commitment). Discussion of these matters in therapy allowed him to discuss these same issues openly with his girlfriend. Although she would have preferred marriage, she was willing to continue in the relationship as it was. Following a heart-to-heart discussion with each other, the couple went on a trip and experienced great sex, including intercourse.

This case is not unusual. We have treated dozens of men who are married or in committed heterosexual relations but have sexual desires for men. These cases differ in terms of the amount and extent of same-sex involvement. Not surprisingly, there are even websites and organizations for married men who are gay. The exact nature of the therapeutic involvement will depend, of course, on the amount of risk, the partner's ability to understand and accept disclosure, the interference and stress the behavior causes, and the misunderstandings associated with the behavior or desires. Not all men choose the path that Mr. Gordon took. His case took a total of 11 sessions over a 9-month period.

Case 7: Mr. and Mrs. Niles (Erectile Disorder and Premature Ejaculation)

Mr. and Mrs. Niles were 71 and 60 years old, respectively; they had been married 10 years when they entered therapy. This was his second marriage and her third. She was a successful singer, with two adult children from her previous marriages. He was a successful businessman, and also had two adult children from his previous marriage. The presenting problem was erectile dysfunction and premature ejaculation. The premature ejaculation was identified as having been a problem since the beginning of the marriage, whereas the erection difficulties had been a problem for 4 years.

Assessment

The assessment interview revealed that despite her extroverted and confident presentation in the entertainment world, at home, Mrs. Niles was unassertive, kept her feelings inside, and had low self-esteem. She assumed that his "rapid" ejaculation and subsequent erection problems occurred because he did not find her attractive and wanted to get the sex act over as quickly as possible or avoid it altogether. She had not discussed her feelings with him, yet she was convinced that she was accurate in these assumptions. She also complained that Mr. Niles was insensitive and controlling. She was now seriously considering divorce and had consulted a lawyer.

He revealed in his assessment interview that he had gone to a urologist and had a RigiScan evaluation. The RigiScan record showed only minimal erection activity, with about 50% rigidity. The urologist told Mr. Niles that, based on his medical history, his problem was vascular. During masturbation, he could achieve a partial erection and ejaculate. Mr. Niles said he loved his wife but noted that she was progressively withdrawing from him, and the more he pressured her for an explanation, the more she withdrew. He acknowledged that he could be insensitive and overbearing at times, although he had recently made some efforts to change. It was his idea to enter therapy. He also noted that she had begun to smoke again (she had quit when they were married) and was drinking more (although not to intoxication). She was unresponsive whenever he attempted to be affectionate or sexual. They had not had sex for 1 year.

Case Formulation and Treatment Plan

This case involved a combination of (1) "premature ejaculation" and (2) generalized, acquired, erectile disorder. Mr. and Mrs. Niles both harbored many sexual and nonsexual misunderstandings that contributed to hurt feelings and emotional distance. Their poor communication skills exacerbated their problems. Mr. Niles's latency to ejaculation was within the normal range on most occasions (2 minutes following intromission), but both Mr. Niles and Mrs. Niles thought that men should be able to control ejaculation for as long as they wished. The erectile dysfunction, more of a problem, was most likely a combination of organic (vasculogenic), interpersonal (nonerotic environment), and intrapersonal (performance anxiety) factors. A strength of the relationship was a foundation of common interests, true admiration, and a strong desire to stay married (especially on Mr. Niles's part). The initial treatment plan consisted of education to dispel misunderstandings, communication training to improve relationship factors, and sensate focus for performance anxiety.

Treatment

When the normality of the ejaculation and the etiology of the erection problems were explained, Mr. and Mrs. Niles showed visible relief. They each accepted responsibility for contributing to miscommunication and agreed to begin therapy by focusing on communication and creating a more positive environment. Mr. Niles asked about Viagra as a solution, and we explained that although this was an option for the future, it was more important for the couple to focus on enjoying each other than on the mechanisms of sex.

Both partners engaged willingly and cooperatively in homework assignments, for example, setting aside time for each other and reading the materials handed out in therapy. Indeed, Mr. Niles made a summary card of effective communication strategies that he carried in his pocket as a reminder! Therapy moved along well and focused on communication and expanded the couple's definition of sex to allow for enjoyable sex without necessarily including intercourse. Viagra, introduced eventually as an adjunct to sex and relationship therapy, helped Mr. Niles to obtain slightly firmer erections that facilitated penetration and relieved him of some residual performance pressure. Within seven therapy sessions, the couple expressed great feelings of success.

This case illustrates that there is often hope despite what might initially appear to be a broken relationship. The key elements for success seemed to be that the problems were caused by correctable misunderstandings, and that the partners were willing to work together and each accept responsibility for change. The total course of therapy took 5 months.

10

Continued Professional
Development and Practice

This chapter is designed to address two questions that you might have at this point: First, how do I obtain further training in sex therapy? And, second, how do I go about starting a sex therapy practice?

Further Training and Continued Development

There are many ways to further your knowledge of sexual health and dysfunction, and to hone your clinical skills. Here, we provide specific suggestions both for the student-in-training (at the postbaccalaureate level) and for the practicing professional (who has already received the terminal degree in his or her discipline). These suggestions are certainly not exhaustive, and we encourage you to be creative as you seek out further training.

Students-in-Training

FIND A MENTOR

For those of you who are still students-in-training, our first piece of advice is to identify a senior-level professional in your discipline with an interest in human sexuality, and to ask that person to serve as your mentor. A mentor can help you to develop efficiently and effectively by providing ongoing research and clinical supervision, by informing you of recent developments in the field

189

(well before these are available in print), and by serving as a role model for your development.

TAKE DIDACTIC COURSES

Regardless of whether you can locate a mentor, you should take didactic courses related to human sexuality. In these days when many universities offer "distance learning," you need not even live near an educational institution. (Of course, we alert you to the potential for charlatans and encourage you to seek out training through accredited institutions.) It is important to emphasize that these courses should not be limited to your academic discipline; that is, if you are a student in a department of psychology, be sure to explore options in both other university departments (e.g., social work, human development, and nursing) and medical schools (e.g., departments of psychiatry, urology, gynecology, and family medicine). Also, be sure to consider courses in the basic sciences, such as anatomy, endocrinology, and physiology. A well-rounded, biopsychosocial background in human sexuality will serve you well.

OBTAIN CLINICAL TRAINING AND EXPERIENCE

If your training program has supervised clinical practica or clerkships that afford experience with the sexual dysfunctions, take them! You might also consider externships and internships that offer specialty tracks in sexuality.

GET INVOLVED IN RESEARCH

Finally, if you are at a research university, a medical center, or a teaching hospital, you can look for opportunities to become involved in sexuality research. Even well-known and internationally recognized scientists welcome volunteer assistants and enjoy nurturing junior colleagues. If you get involved with a research team, you will probably have the chance to present findings at local, national, or international meetings and conventions.

Establishing a Foundation of Knowledge

We advise that all health practitioners, regardless of their professional training as therapists or physicians, obtain a basic knowledge of human sexuality. Questions about sexual development, paraphilia, sexual orientation, gender identity, and sexual trauma are just a sampling of the concerns of patients presenting with sexual dysfunction. There are a number of complementary ways to achieve such a foundation.

READ AN INTRODUCTORY-LEVEL, COLLEGE TEXTBOOK

An efficient way to gain a broad and well-rounded perspective on human sexuality and recent research is to read one of the many fine human sexuality textbooks now available. One that we have found useful is Crooks and Baur's (1999), *Our Sexuality*. This sensitive, comprehensive, well-written text is an excellent resource to have in one's office. There are many other fine textbooks available from most of the major academic publishing houses. We would advise that you read a recent book, however, because of the rapidly changing knowledge about human sexuality, sexual dysfunctions, and HIV and other STDs.

READ THE "CLASSICS"

Another valuable way to obtain foundation knowledge (and a sense of the history of the field) is to read the classic works in the field, such as the following:

Kaplan, H. S. (1974). *The new sex therapy.* New York: Brunner/Mazel.
Masters, W. H., & Johnson, V. E. (1966). *Human sexual response.* Boston: Little, Brown.
Masters, W. H., & Johnson V. E. (1970). *Human sexual inadequacy.* Boston: Little, Brown.

READ RECENT SCIENTIFIC BOOKS ON HUMAN SEXUALITY

The following "soon-to-be-classics" also provide current and useful information:

Laumann, E. O., Gagnon, J. H., Michael, R. T., & Michaels, S. (1994). *The social organization of sexuality: Sexual practices in the United States.* Chicago: University of Chicago.
Leiblum, S. R., & Rosen, R. C. (Eds.). (2000). *Principles and practice of sex therapy* (3rd ed.). New York: Guilford.
Rosen, R. C., & Leiblum, S. R. (Eds.). (1995). *Case studies in sex therapy.* New York: Guilford.
Zilbergeld, B. (1999). *The new male sexuality* (rev. ed.). New York: Bantam.

STAY ABREAST OF CURRENT DEVELOPMENTS BY READING PROFESSIONAL JOURNALS

In addition to reading the "classic" professional books, we encourage you to stay current by subscribing to and reading (this is the harder part!) some or all of the following journals:

Archives of Sexual Behavior—published by Kluwer Academic Publishers, 101 Philip Drive, Assinippi Park, Norwell, MA 02061; *www.wkap.nl/journalhome.htm/ 0004-0002*

Journal of Psychology and Human Sexuality—published by Haworth Press, 10 Alice Street, Binghamton, NY 13904-1580; *www.haworthpressinc.com/Home.htm*

Journal of Sex Education and Therapy—published by the American Association of Sex Educators, Counselors, and Therapists, Inc. (see below), Suite 2-A, 103 Avenue South, Mount Vernon, IA 52314; *www.aasect.org/jset.cfm*

Journal of Sex Research—published by the Society for the Scientific Study of Sexuality (see below), P.O. Box 416, Allentown, PA 18105-0416; *www.ssc.wisc.edu/ ssss/index.html*

Journal of Sex and Marital Therapy—published by Brunner–Routledge, 325 Chestnut Street, Suite 800, Philadelphia, PA 19106; *www.taylorandfrancis.com/JNLS/ smt.htm*

JOIN PROFESSIONAL ORGANIZATIONS DEVOTED TO RESEARCH ON HUMAN SEXUALITY

It is a good idea to join at least one of the many professional organizations devoted to the dissemination of recent information about sexuality. Among the most well-known organizations are the following:

The American Association of Sex Educators, Counselors, and Therapists (AASECT) is devoted to the promotion of sexual health by the development and advancement of the fields of sex therapy, counseling, and education. Its mission is to provide professional education and certification of sex educators, counselors, and therapists, as well as individuals who supervise sex therapists in training. AASECT also encourages research related to sex education, counseling, and therapy, and supports the publication and dissemination of professional materials related to these fields. To achieve its mission, AASECT offers a broad range of professional education and training activities, including a certification program, an annual meeting, and the *Journal of Sex Education and Therapy*. For information write to AASECT, Suite 2-A, 103 Avenue South, Mount Vernon, IA 52314 (*www.aasect.org/jset.cfm*).

The Society for the Scientific Study of Sexuality (SSSS) is an international organization dedicated to the advancement of knowledge about sexuality. It is the oldest organization of professionals interested in the study of sexuality in the United States. SSSS brings together an interdisciplinary group of professionals who believe in the importance of both the production of quality research and the clinical, educational, and social applications of research related to all aspects of sexuality. It holds an annual meeting and publishes the *Journal of Sex Research*. Membership information can be obtained by writing to SSSS at P.O. Box 416, Allentown, PA 18105-0416 (*www.ssc.wisc.edu/ssss/ index.html*).

The International Academy of Sex Researchers (IASR) is the most exclusive professional organization. IASR is a scientific society whose objective is the promotion of high standards of research and scholarship in the field of sexual behavior by fostering communication and cooperation among scholars engaged in such research. Membership is contingent upon scientific productivity in the field. IASR holds an annual meeting (which alternates between the United States and other countries) and publishes the journal *Archives of Sexual Behavior.* Membership information can be obtained by writing to Kenneth J. Zucker, PhD, Secretary/Treasurer, International Academy of Sex Research, Child Psychiatry Program, Centre for Addiction and Mental Health—Clarke Division, 250 College Street, Toronto, Ontario M5T 1R8, Canada.

The Society for Sex Therapy and Research (SSTAR), which began as an informal coalition of sex therapists primarily associated with medical schools in the northeastern United States, has subsequently expanded its membership and society goals. Currently, SSTAR represents a community of professionals who have clinical or research interests in human sexual concerns. Its goals are to facilitate communications among clinicians who treat problems of sexual identity, sexual function, and reproductive life, and provide a forum for exchange of ideas between those interested in research in human sexuality and those whose primary activities are patient care. These goals are accomplished by an annual meeting and, occasionally, a smaller, regional meeting or publication of a special document. The membership is multidisciplinary, with the criterion that members be actively involved in treatment or clinical investigation of sexual disorders and possess superior clinical competence and high ethical standards. The membership includes professionals in varying disciplines including social work, nursing, physiology, gynecology, urology, internal medicine, psychiatry, and psychology. This permits an interaction between people of diverse disciplines, allowing each to contribute his or her unique perspective. Further information can be obtained by writing to the Society at 409 12th Street, SW, P.O. Box 96920, Washington, DC 20090-6920 (*www.sstarnet.org*).

Memberships in these societies will make it easier for you to attend conventions and enroll in workshops. In addition, through their publications, you will find it easier to follow current developments in the field.

SEEK POSTDOCTORAL TRAINING

If your life situation will allow you to make less money, and to live in another city for a year or two, you might seek more formalized training experiences. For example, you might consider supervised externships and postdoctoral training opportunities that are increasingly available in major cities and can be located through professional publications such as the American Psychological Association's *Monitor.*

Starting a Sex Therapy Practice

The purpose of this section is to provide some guidelines for setting up a successful private practice that focuses on the assessment and treatment of sexual dysfunctions. Although we touch upon aspects of professional practice that may be classified as entrepreneurial, our primary goal is to discuss the components of professional practice that are unique to the specialty area of the sexual dysfunctions. Our belief is that the nitty-gritty of business, such as whether to rent or buy your office, how to hire support personnel, and what office equipment to select, can be addressed better in other sources. Therefore, we turn our attention to the following issues: certification and licensure, client recruitment, insurance reimbursement, and ethics.

Licensure and Certification: What's in a Name?

Licensing is legislation that protects and defines the role and duties of a therapist; certification legislation protects professional titles. To our knowledge, however, there are no states that grant a specific licensure or certification for "sex therapist." Those professionals who call themselves sex therapists and who claim to be licensed or certified by a state board of professional regulations are usually licensed in a core discipline, such as psychology, social work, medicine, or nursing. As a result of the absence of state licensing or certification, it is possible for anyone to present him- or herself as a sex therapist without any credentials, training, or expertise.

AASECT (mentioned earlier) does offer a certification program. To be eligible, a professional needs to have a master's degree plus 3 years of professional experience in the field, or a doctorate, with 2 years of experience. In addition, the therapist must also have completed 150 hours of sex therapy supervised by an AASECT-certified therapist. Although a reasonable program, the AASECT certification procedure is not regulated on a state level, is not required for practice, and is not recognized by most consumers. Not surprisingly, then, there are many excellent sex therapists who do not take the trouble to obtain this certification.

In addition to the matter of licensing and/or certification, there is the related matter of what one should call oneself professionally (e.g., how to list oneself in the telephone directory). This is not a trivial matter. Consider for example, the following experience. One of us (JPW) was recently called upon as an "expert" witness to give testimony in a criminal case regarding a sexual offense. The opposing attorney did his homework and attempted to disallow the testimony on the grounds that he was "merely a sex therapist" and not a professional expert. When it was demonstrated that the witness was a "licensed PhD clinical psychologist," who happened to have expertise in human sexuality, the testimony was allowed. A subsequent, informal survey of colleagues from across the country indicated that one earns more professional credibility by titling oneself in terms of primary professional training rather than as a "sex therapist."

Patient Recruitment

One's title may affect patient recruitment, although we know of no research that has addressed this issue. For example, regarding telephone directory listings, our impression is that these listings result in few if any direct referrals. It seems that telephone listings are most useful to current clients and colleagues who have forgotten our number! Instead, there seem to be two excellent sources of client referrals: other professionals (especially physicians) and satisfied clients. Because there is not much one can do, for ethical reasons, to enhance client-based referrals, we recommend the "other professionals" route.

Several strategies seem to be effective in alerting other professionals to your expertise, the clinical services you offer, and so on. First, a method that appears very useful is to give free talks to professional organizations, such as local primary care or family practice physicians. Of course, it is important that you gear your talk (vocabulary and content) to your audience, and that you be well prepared. A second method would be to provide in-service training to local practitioners, trainees, and clinics. In this way, you become known as a person who is comfortable and skilled in dealing with sexual dysfunctions. Third, once you are experienced, and only after you are very adept at handling difficult questions, you might try carefully selected interviews with the local news media (print and electronic). This can be slippery and dangerous ground though, so beware! Finally, we have found that publishing research findings generates referrals from outside our local areas. So if you have an opportunity to do research, or to collaborate with other colleagues on research, you may find that this provides some dividends in terms of clients. Moreover, involvement in research is stimulating and challenging in its own right.

It is also important to establish links with other professionals, so that you will be able to provide the highest-quality care. In our view, the clinical practices that serve clients best are those multidisciplinary services that aim to incorporate the latest biopsychosocial and technical advances in assessment and treatment. These practices tend to be associated with teaching-hospitals and university clinics. If you are not a part of such a setting, you will have to organize a collaborative effort with other professionals in order to offer your clients comprehensive care.

To establish such a team, you should try to develop a working collaboration with professionals having several medical specialties: urologists, gynecologists, and endocrinologists. The urologist should be familiar with the comprehensive assessment, diagnosis, and treatment of male sexual complaints. Preferably, the urologist will be sensitive to psychosocial contributions to sexual dysfunctions and not just interested in biomedical solutions. A gynecologist is invaluable for the assessment of female disorders. Like urologists, gynecologists vary widely in their knowledge of and sensitivity to sexual problems. It is a positive sign if the gynecologist and urologist with whom you work recognize that the restoration of intercourse is not the only goal in helping clients with sexual problems. Finally, the last "core" physician is the endocrinologist, who will be needed to complete hormonal evaluations and to monitor hormone therapy when this is indicated. Also, because endocrinologists tend to be well informed about diabetes, a common precipitating cause of sexual dysfunction in men and women, it is very helpful to have a colleague in this area.

In addition to this "core" group, you will occasionally need to consult with a cardiologist (regarding the effects of hypertension, antihypertensive medications, and the effects of various forms of cardiac illness), a neurologist (regarding the influence of seizure disorders and other neurological problems upon sexual function), and an infectious disease specialist (regarding AIDS and other STDs). Finally, because there is always the need for general medical screening, it is good to know an internist or family practitioner to whom you can refer. Also, such "medical generalists" often need psychosocial colleagues to whom to refer their patients, so they can be a good source of referrals.

We believe that it is feasible to be in private practice and to treat sexual problems. However, if this is your situation, we strongly encourage you to establish the kind of referral network or comprehensive team described earlier. To work without such collaboration and consultation, in our view, teeters dangerously close to the kind of professional "know-it-all-ism" that might lead to malpractice. Besides, it can be professionally lonely!

Insurance Reimbursement

Health care insurance, especially so-called "mental" health care insurance, continues to be a nightmare—not just for sex therapy, but for all psychotherapies. Every practitioner has his or her horror stories to tell, and we are no different. Given the plethora of coverages, companies, and plans, it is difficult to provide a global statement. However, in our experience, most insurance companies do not reimburse for treatment if the recorded diagnosis is a sexual dysfunction. A diagnosis of depression or anxiety disorder may be justifiable and is reimbursable.

Ethics and Sex Therapy

We have previously described the absence of state-regulated licensing and/or certification. Perhaps it is true that part of the reason why such formal recognition is absent is that there is skepticism associated with the "sex therapist" label. The general public, and elected officials who represent them, may still be affected by the bad press associated with sex therapists during the 1960s and early 1970s. In a thoughtful text published by the Walk-In Counseling Center of Minneapolis, Schoener, Milgrom, Gonsiorek, Luepker, and Conroe (1990) point out that the human potential movement of the 1960s resulted in considerable experimentation with types and practices of psychotherapy. Specifically, there were articles published in professional journals and presentations made at professional meetings that advocated the use of bizarre and unethical practices such as nude marathon sessions with clients; touching, hugging, kissing, and sexual intercourse with clients. Although the advocates of these unethical approaches were in the minority, the popular press magnified their message. Thus, a widespread impression of sex therapists as "flaky perverts" was created. Unfortunately, these impressions are still with us, and they are in the minds of some patients who enter therapy.

Because of this history, those who practice sex therapy today have to be impeccable professionals. Not only should we abide by the ethical standards of our professions, but we must also avoid even the appearance of impropriety. Although we do not have the space to elaborate upon all ethical violations that are to be avoided, we wish to mention the most important ones.

You must absolutely avoid sexual intimacies with clients and observe appropriate professional boundaries in your work. Because therapy inevitably places patients in a vulnerable position and creates a psychological dependence upon the therapist, a power differential exists that creates a potential for sexual victimization. In addition to the usual factors that contribute to patient vulnerability, the explicit discussion of intimate sexual material increases the potential for transference and countertransference to occur. Moreover, many persons who seek treatment for sexual dysfunctions have had a history of sexual abuse; these persons appear to be at increased risk of being revictimized by others, even therapists (Broden & Agresti, 1998). For these reasons, you must be especially sensitive to patient welfare. You should establish professional policies that ensure against crossing the well-established and important boundaries that have been established.

Most professionals quickly dismiss this matter as not applying to them. However, surveys suggest that the prevalence of sexual abuse of patients by professionals (i.e., physicians, psychologists, social workers, and pastoral counselors) ranges from 3% to 18% (e.g., Holroyd & Brodsky, 1977); that is, 3–18% of those surveyed have admitted to having sexual contact with their clients on at least one occasion. Schoener et al. (1990) remind us that the single, most frequent basis for a malpractice suit against psychologists is sexual malpractice. Similarly, in a 1985 survey of social workers, the leading cause of legal claims was sexual contact with clients (Besharov, 1985). Furthermore, indirect evidence for the continuing problem comes from the state legislatures.

Laws regulating the sexual misconduct of therapists fall into four categories: civil, criminal, reporting, and injunctive relief statutes. The theoretical underpinnings of the various laws, an overview of the advantages and disadvantages of each category, and the laws as they exist in various states are reviewed in an article by Haspel, Jorgenson, Wincze, and Parsons (1997).

Concluding Comments

In this book, we have tried to present a first course in the assessment and treatment of sexual dysfunctions. In conjunction with supervised clinical training and experience, we hope that this book will help you to feel comfortable about and prepared to address the sexual difficulties of your clients. Moreover, we have broached many topics that we hope you will have found intriguing and that might encourage further study.

In the course of providing sex assessment and therapy, we have been impressed by the grateful responses of our patients. Many report that they are expressing their sexual concerns and secrets for the first time. This opportunity to discuss sexual matters openly and without shame can be therapeutic for many patients. Even more gratifying are those moments when, through the straightforward therapeutic approach described in this book, we can help our patients to reestablish sexual functioning, health, and satisfaction. We wish you many similar moments.

References

Abarbanel, A. (1978). Diagnosis and treatment of coital discomfort. In J. LoPiccolo & L. LoPiccolo (Eds.), *Handbook of sex therapy* (pp. 241–259). New York: Plenum.

American Psychological Association. (1987). *Casebook on ethical principles of psychologists.* Washington, DC: Author.

American Psychiatric Association. (2000). *Diagnostic and statistical manual of mental disorders* (4th ed., Text Revision). Washington, DC: Author.

Apfelbaum, B. (2000). Retarded ejaculation: A much misunderstood syndrome. In S. R. Leiblum & R. C. Rosen (Eds.), *Principles and practice of sex therapy* (3rd ed., pp. 205–241). New York: Guilford.

Ard, B. N., Jr. (1977). Sex in lasting marriages: A longitudinal study. *Journal of Sex Research, 13,* 274–285.

Ashton, A. K. (1999). Sildenafil treatment of paroxetine-induced anorgasmia in a woman. *American Journal of Psychiatry, 156,* 800.

Assalian, P. (1988). Clomipramine in the treatment of premature ejaculation. *Journal of Sex Research, 24,* 213–215.

Athanasiou, R., Shaver, P., & Tavris, C. (1970, July). Sex. *Psychology Today,* pp. 39–51.

Baggaley, M. R., Hirst, J. F., & Watson, J. P. (1996). Outcome of patients referred to a psychosexual clinic with erectile failure. *Sexual and Marital Therapy, 11,* 123–130.

Balko, A., Malhotra, C., Wincze, J., Susset, J., Bansal, S., Carney, W., & Hopkins, R. (1986). Deep penile vein arterialization for arterial and venous impotence. *Archives of Surgery, 121,* 774–777.

Balon, R. (1996). Antidepressants in the treatment of premature ejaculation. *Journal of Sex and Marital Therapy, 22,* 85–96.

Bancroft, J. (1984). Hormones and human sexual behavior. *Journal of Sex and Marital Therapy, 10,* 3–21.

Bancroft, J. (1988). Sexual desire and the brain. *Sexual and Marital Therapy, 3,* 11–27.

Bancroft, J. (1989). *Human sexuality and its problems* (2nd ed.). Edinburgh, Scotland: Churchill Livingstone.

Bancroft, J., & Coles, L. (1976). Three years' experience in a sexual problems clinic. *British Medical Journal, 1,* 1575–1577.

Bancroft, J., & Wu, F. (1983). Changes in erectile responsiveness during androgen replacement therapy. *Archives of Sexual Behavior, 12,* 59–66.

Bandura, A. (1997). *Self-efficacy: The exercise of control.* New York: Freeman.

Bansal, S. (1988). Sexual dysfunction in hypertensive men: A critical review of the literature. *Hypertension, 12,* 1–10.

Barlow, D. H. (1986). Causes of sexual dysfunction: The role of anxiety and cognitive interference. *Journal of Consulting and Clinical Psychology, 54,* 140–148.

Barlow, D. H. (1988). *Anxiety and its disorders: The nature and treatment of anxiety and panic.* New York: Guilford.

Barlow, D. H., Cardozo, L. D., Francis, R. M., Griffin, M., Hart, D. M., Stephens, E., & Sturdee, D. W. (1997). Urogenital aging and its effect on sexual health in older British women. *British Journal of Obstetrics and Gynecology, 104,* 87–91.

Barlow, D. H., Hayes, S. C., & Nelson, R. 0. (1984). *The scientist–practitioner: Research and accountability in clinical and educational settings.* Elmsford, NY: Pergamon.

Barlow, D. H., Sakheim, D., & Beck, J. G. (1983). Anxiety increases sexual arousal. *Journal of Abnormal Psychology, 92,* 49–54.

Barnes, J. (1981). Non-consummation of marriage. *Irish Medical Journal, 74,* 19–21.

Barnes, J. (1986a). Primary vaginismus (Part 1): Social and clinical features. *Irish Medical Journal, 79,* 59–62.

Barnes, J. (1986b). Primary vaginismus (Part 2): Aetiological factors. *Irish Medical Journal, 79,* 62–65.

Bartlik, B., & Goldberg, J. (2000). Female sexual arousal disorder. In S. R. Leiblum & R. C. Rosen (Eds.), *Principles and practice of sex therapy* (3rd ed., pp. 85–117). New York: Guilford.

Bartlik, B., Kaplan, P. & Kaplan, H. (1995). Psychostimulants apparently reverse sexual dysfunction secondary to selective serotonin re-uptake inhibitors. *Journal of Sex and Marital Therapy, 21,* 264–271.

Bartlik, B., Legere, R., & Andersson, L. (1999). The combined use of sex therapy and testosterone replacement therapy for women. *Psychiatric Annals, 29,* 27–33.

Beck, A. T. (1976). *Cognitive therapy and the emotional disorders.* New York: International Universities.

Beck, A. T. (1988). *Love is never enough.* New York: Harper & Row.

Beck, J. G. (1995). Hypoactive sexual desire disorder: An overview. *Journal of Consulting and Clinical Psychology, 65,* 919–927.

Beck, J. G., Barlow, D. H., & Sakheim, D. (1983). The effects of attentional focus and partner arousal on sexual responding in functional and dysfunctional men. *Behaviour Research and Therapy, 21,* 1–8.

Becker, J. V. (1989). Impact of sexual abuse on sexual functioning. In S. R. Leiblum & R. C. Rosen (Eds.), *Principles and practice of sex therapy* (2nd ed.): *Update for the 1990s* (pp. 298–318). New York: Guilford.

Beers, M. H., & Berkow, R. (Eds.). (1999). *The Merck manual of diagnosis and therapy* (17th ed.). Rahway, NJ: Merck.

Beggs, V. E., Calhoun, K. S., & Wolchik, S. A. (1987). Sexual anxiety and female sexual arousal: A comparison of arousal during sexual anxiety stimuli and sexual pleasure stimuli. *Archives of Sexual Behavior, 16,* 311–319.

Behrendt, A. E., & George, K. D. (1995). Sex therapy for gay and bisexual men. In L. Diamant & R. D. McAnulty (Eds.), *The psychology of sexual orientation, behavior, and identity: A handbook* (pp. 220–236). Wesport, CT: Greenwood Press.

Beitchman, J. H., Zucker, K. J., Hood, J. E., daCosta, G. A., Akman, D., & Cassavia, E. (1992). A review of the long-term effects of child sexual abuse. *Child Abuse and Neglect, 16,* 101–118.

Bennett, A. H. (1988). Venous arterialization for erectile impotence. *Urologic Clinics of North America, 15,* 111–113.

Benson, G. (1994). Endocrine factors related to impotence. In A. Bennett (Ed.), *Impotence: Diagnosis and management of erectile dysfunction* (pp. 31–41). Philadelphia: Saunders.

Bergeron, S., Binik, Y. M., Khalifé, S., Meana, M., Berkley, K. J., & Pagidas, K. (1997). The treatment of vulvar vestibulitis syndrome: Towards a multimodal approach. *Sexual and Marital Therapy, 12,* 305–311.

Bergeron, S., Bouchard C., Fortier M., Binik Y. M., & Khalifé, S. (1997). The surgical treatment of vulvar vestibulitis syndrome: A follow-up study. *Journal of Sex and Marital Therapy, 23,* 317–325.

Besharov, D. J. (1985). *The vulnerable social worker: Liability for serving children and families.* Silver Springs, MD: National Association of Social Workers.

Bhui, K., Herriot, P., Dein, S., & Watson, J. P. (1994). Asians presenting to a sex and marital therapy clinic. *International Journal of Social Psychiatry, 40,* 194–204.

Bhui, K., Puffet, A., & Strathdee, G. (1997). Sexual and relationship problems amongst patients with severe chronic psychoses. *Social Psychiatry and Psychiatric Epidemiology, 32,* 459–467.

Binik, Y. M., Bergeron, S., & Khalifé, S. (2000). Dyspareunia. In S. R. Leiblum & R. C. Rosen (Eds.), *Principles and practice of sex therapy* (3rd ed., pp. 154–180). New York: Guilford.

Bornstein, J., Goldik, Z., Stolar, Z., Zarfati, D., & Abramovici, H. (1997). Predicting the outcome of surgical treatment of vulvar vestibulitis. *Obstetrics and Gynecology, 89,* 695–698.

Bradford, J. (1997). Medical interventions in sexual deviance. In D. R. Laws & W. O'Donohue (Eds.) *Sexual deviance: Theory, assessment, and treatment* (pp. 449–464). New York: Guilford.

Brindley, G. (1983). Cavernosal alpha-blockade: A new technique for investigating and treating erectile impotence. *British Journal of Psychiatry, 143,* 332–337.

Broden, M. S., & Agresti, A. A. (1998). Responding to therapists' sexual abuse of adult incest survivors: Ethical and legal considerations. *Psychotherapy, 35,* 96–104.

Broekman, C., Haensel, S., Van de Ven, L., & Slob, A. (1992). Bisoprolol and hypertension: Effects on sexual functioning in men. *Journal of Sex and Marital Therapy, 18,* 325–331.

Buffum, J. (1986). Pharmacosexology update: Prescription drugs and sexual function. *Journal of Psychoactive Drugs, 18,* 97–106.

Burnap, D. W., & Golden, J. S. (1967). Sexual problems in medical practice. *Journal of Medical Education, 42,* 673–680.

Cacioppo, J. T., & Tassinary, L. G. (1990). Inferring psychological significance from physiological signals. *American Psychologist, 45,* 16–28.

Caird, W., & Wincze, J. P. (1977). *Sex therapy: A behavioral approach.* New York: Harper & Row.

Carani, C., Zini, D., Baldini, A., Della Casa, L., Ghizzani, A., & Marrama, P. (1990). Effects of androgen treatment in impotent men with normal and low levels of free testosterone. *Archives of Sexual Behavior, 19,* 223–234.

Carey, M. P. (1999). Prevention of HIV infection through changes in sexual behavior. *American Journal of Health Promotion, 14,* 104–111.

Carey, M. P., Braaten, L. S., Maisto, S. A., Gleason, J. R., Forsyth, A. D., Durant, L. E., & Jaworski, B. C. (2000). Using information, motivational enhancement, and skills training to reduce the risk of HIV infection for low-income urban women: A second randomized clinical trial. *Health Psychology, 19,* 3–11.

Carey, M. P., Flasher, L. V., Maisto, S. A., & Turkat, I. D. (1984). The a priori approach to psychological assessment. *Professional Psychology: Research and Practice, 15,* 515–527.

Carey, M. P., & Johnson, B. T. (1996). Effectiveness of yohimbine in the treatment of erectile disorder: Four meta-analytic integrations. *Archives of Sexual Behavior, 25,* 341–360.

Carey, M. P., Maisto, S. A., Kalichman, S. C., Forsyth, A. D., Wright, E. M., & Johnson, B. T. (1997). Enhancing motivation to reduce the risk of HIV infection for economically disadvantaged urban women. *Journal of Consulting and Clinical Psychology, 65,* 531–541.

Carey, M. P., Morrison-Beedy, D., & Johnson, B. T. (1997). The HIV-Knowledge Questionnaire: Development and evaluation of a reliable, valid, and practical self-administered questionnaire. *AIDS and Behavior, 1,* 61–74.

Carson, C., Kirby, R., & Goldstein, I. (Eds.). (1999). *Textbook of erectile dysfunction.* Oxford, UK: Isis Medical Media.

Catalan, J., Klimes, I., Bond, A., Day, A., Garrod, A., & Rizza, C. (1992a). The psychosocial impact of HIV infection in men with haemophilia: Controlled investigation and factors associated with psychiatric morbidity. *Journal of Psychosomatic Research, 36,* 409–416.

Catalan, J., Klimes, I., Day, A., Garrod, A., Bond, A., & Gallwey, J. (1992b). The psychosocial impact of HIV infection in gay men: A controlled investigation and factors associated with psychiatric morbidity. *British Journal of Psychiatry, 161,* 774–778.

Chambless, D. L., Stem, T., Sultan, F. E., Williams, A. J., Goldstein, A. J., Lineberger, M. H., Lifshitz, J. L., & Kelly, L. (1982). The pubococcygens and female orgasm: A correlational study with normal subjects. *Archives of Sexual Behavior, 11,* 479–490.

Chambless, D. L., Sultan, F. E., Stem, T. E., O'Neill, C., Garrison, S., & Jackson, A.

(1984). Effect of pubococcygeal exercise on coital orgasm in women. *Journal of Consulting and Clinical Psychology, 52,* 114–118.

Chandraiah, S., Levenson, J. L., & Collins, J. B. (1991). Sexual dysfunction, social maladjustment, and psychiatric disorders in women seeking treatment in a premenstrual syndrome clinic. *International Journal of Psychiatry in Medicine, 21,* 189–204.

Cogen, R., & Steinman, W. (1990). Sexual function and practice in elderly men of low socioeconpmic status. *Journal of Family Practice, 31,* 162–166.

Cole, W. G. (1956). *Sex in Christianity and psychoanalysis.* London: Allen & Unwin.

Coleman, E. (1987). Sexual compulsivity: Definition, etiology, and treatment considerations. In E. Coleman (Ed.), *Chemical dependency and intimacy dysfunction* (pp. 189–204). New York: Haworth.

Coleman, E. (1990). The obsessive–compulsive model for describing compulsive sexual behavior. *American Journal of Preventive Psychiatry and Neurology, 2,* 9–14.

Coleman, E., & Rosser, B. R. S. (1996). Gay and bisexual male sexuality. In R. P. Cabaj & T. S. Stein (Eds.), *Textbook of homosexuality and mental health* (pp. 707–721). Washington, DC: American Psychiatric Press.

Comfort, A. (1998). *The new joy of sex and more joy of sex.* New York: Simon & Schuster.

Conte, H. R. (1986). Multivariate assessment of sexual dysfunction. *Journal of Consulting and Clinical Psychology, 5,* 149–157.

Cooper, A. J. (1994). The effects of intoxication levels of ethanol on nocturnal penile tumescence. *Journal of Sex and Marital Therapy, 20,* 14–23.

Cozby, P. C. (1973). Self-disclosure: A literature review. *Psychological Bulletin, 79,* 73–91.

Crenshaw, T., & Goldberg, J. (1996). *Sexual Pharmacology.* New York: Norton.

Crooks, R. L., & Baur, K. (1999). *Our sexuality* (7th ed.). Belmont, CA: Wadsworth.

Damrav, F. (1963). Premature ejaculation: Use of ethyl amino benzoate to prolong coitus. *Journal of Urology, 89,* 936–939.

Davidson, J. M., Camargo, C. A., Smith, E. R., & Kwan, M. (1983). Maintenance of sexual function in a castrated man treated with ovarian steroids. *Archives of Sexual Behavior, 12,* 263–274.

Davis, C. M., Yarber, W. L., Bauserman, R., Schreer, G., & Davis, S. L. (Eds.). (1998). *Handbook of sexually-related measures.* Thousand Oaks, CA: Sage.

Delizonna, L. L., Wincze, J. P., Litz, B. T., Brown, T. A., & Barlow, D. H. (2001). A comparison of subjective and physiological measures of mechanically produced and erotically produced erections: Or, is an erection an erection? *Journal of Sex and Marital Therapy, 27,* 21–31.

Derogatis, L. R. (1975). *Derogatis Sexual Functioning Inventory (DSFI): Preliminary scoring manual.* Baltimore: Clinical Psychometric Research.

Derogatis, L. R., Fagan, P. J., Schmidt, C. W., Wise, T. N., & Gilden, K. S. (1986). Psychological subtypes of anorgasmia: A marker variable approach. *Journal of Sex and Marital Therapy, 12,* 197–210.

Derogatis, L. R., & Melisaratos, N. (1979). The DSFI: A multidimensional measure of sexual functioning. *Journal of Sex and Marital Therapy, 5,* 244–281.

Derogatis, L. R., & Meyer, J. K. (1979). A psychological profile of the sexual dysfunctions. *Archives of Sexual Behavior, 8,* 201–223.

Derogatis, L. R., Meyer, J. K., & King, K. M. (1981). Psychopathology in individuals with sexual dysfunction. *American Journal of Psychiatry, 138,* 757–763.

Derogatis, L. R., & Spencer, P. M. (1982). *The Brief Symptom Inventory (BSI): Administration, scoring, and procedures manual—I.* Baltimore: Clinical Psychometric Research.

Derouet, H., Caspari, D., Rohde, V., Rommel, G., & Ziegler, M. (1999). Treatment of erectile dysfunction with external vacuum devices. *Andrologia, 31*(Suppl. 1), 89–94.

de Silva, P., & Todd, G. (1998). Sexual dysfunction in women with anorexia nervosa: Nature and treatment. *Journal of Sex and Marital Therapy, 13,* 21–36.

Diokno, A. C., Brown, M. B., & Herzog, A. R. (1990). Sexual function in the elderly. *Archives of Internal Medicine, 150,* 197–200.

Dove, N. L., & Wiederman, M. W. (2000). Cognitive distraction and women's sexual functioning. *Journal of Sex and Marital Therapy, 26,* 67–78.

Duddle, C. M. (1977). Etiological factors in the unconsummated marriage. *Journal of Psychosomatic Research, 21,* 157–160.

Dunn, K. M., Croft, P. R., & Hackett, G. I. (1999). Association pf sexual problems with social, psychological and physical problems in men and women: A cross sectional population survey. *Journal of Epidemiology and Community Health, 53,* 144–148.

Dunn, M. E., & Trost, J. E. (1989). Male multiple orgasms: A descriptive study. *Archives of Sexual Behavior, 18,* 377–387.

Earle C. M., Seah, M., Coulden, S. E., Stuckey, B. G., & Keogh, E. J. (1996). The use of the vacuum erection device in the management of erectile impotence. *International Journal of Impotence Research, 8,* 237–240.

Ellis, A. (1962). *Reason and emotion in psychotherapy.* New York: Lyle Stuart.

Ellis, H. (1906). *Studies in the psychology of sex* (7 vols.). New York: Random House.

El-Rufaie, O. E. F., Bener, A., Abuzeid, M. S. O., & Ali, T. A. (1997). Sexual dysfunction among type II diabetic men: A controlled study. *Journal of Psychosomatic Medicine, 43,* 605–613.

Engel, G. L. (1977). The need for a new medical model: A challenge for biomedicine. *Science, 196,* 129–136.

Ernst, C., Foeldenyi, M., & Angst, J. (1993). The Zurich study: XXI. Sexual dysfunctions and disturbances in young adults: Data of a longitudinal epidemiological study. *European Archives of Psychiatry and Clinical Neuroscience, 243,* 179–188.

Ertekin, C. (1998). Diabetes mellitus and sexual dysfunction. *Scandinavian Journal of Sexology, 1,* 3–22.

Exner, J. E., Jr. (1986). *The Rorschach: A comprehensive system: Vol. 1. Basic foundations* (2nd ed.). New York: Wiley.

Fahrner, E.-M. (1987). Sexual dysfunction in male alcohol addicts: Prevalence and treatment. *Archives of Sexual Behavior, 16,* 247–257.

Fass, R., Fullerton, S., Naliboff, B., Hirsh, T., & Mayer, E. A. (1998). Sexual dysfunction in patients with irritable bowel syndrome and non-ulcer dyspepsia. *Digestion, 59,* 79–85.

Fassinger, R. E., & Morrow, S. L. (1995). Overcome: Repositioning lesbian sexualities. In L. Diamant & R. D. McAnulty (Eds.), *The psychology of sexual orientation, behavior, and identity: A handbook* (pp. 197–219). Wesport, CT: Greenwood.

Feldman, H. A., Goldstein, I., Hatzichristou, D. G., Krane, R. J., & McKinlay, J. B. (1994). Impotence and its medical and psychosocial correlates: Results of the Massachusetts Male Aging Study. *Journal of Urology, 151,* 54–61.

Fisher, J., & Corcoran, K. J. (1994a). *Measures for clinical practice: A sourcebook: Vol. 1. Couples, families, and children* (2nd ed.). New York: Free Press.

Fisher, J., & Corcoran, K. J. (1994b). *Measures for clinical practice: A sourcebook: Vol. 2. Adults* (2nd ed.). New York: Free Press.

Fisher, J. D., & Fisher, W. A. (1992). Changing AIDS-risk behavior. *Psychological Bulletin, 111,* 455–474.

Fisher, S. (1973). *The female orgasm.* New York: Basic Books.

Fisher, W. A. (1988). The Sexual Opinion Survey. In C. M. Davis, W. L. Yarber, & S. L. Davis (Eds.), *Sexuality-related measures: A compendium* (pp. 34–37). Lake Mills, IA: Graphic.

Fisher, W. A., Byrne, D., White, L. A., & Kelley, K. (1988). Erotophobia–erotophilia as a dimension of personality. *Journal of Sex Research, 25,* 123–151.

Fisher, W. A., & Fisher, J. D. (1998). Understanding and promoting sexual and reproductive health behavior: Theory and method. *Annual Review of Sex Research, 9,* 39–76.

Frank, E., Anderson, C., & Kupfer, D. J. (1976). Profiles of couples seeking sex therapy and marital therapy. *American Journal of Psychiatry, 133,* 559–562.

Frank, E., Anderson, C., & Rubinstein, D. (1978). Frequency of sexual dysfunction in "normal" couples. *New England Journal of Medicine, 299,* 111–115.

Friedman, R. C., & Downey, J. I. (1994). Homosexuality. *New England Journal of Medicine, 331,* 923–930.

Fugl-Meyer, A.R., & Sjogren Fugl-Meyer, K. (1999). Sexual disabilities, problems, and satisfaction in 18–74 year old Swedes. *Scandanavian Journal of Sexology, 3,* 79–105.

Gagnon, J. H. (1977). *Human sexualities.* Glenview, IL: Scott, Foresman.

Gangakhedkar, R. R., Bentley, M. E., Divekar, A. D., Gadkari, D., Mehendale, S. M., Shepherd, M. E., Bollinger, R. C., & Quinn, T. C. (1997). Spread of HIV infection in married monogamous women in India. *Journal of the American Medical Association, 278,* 2090–2092.

Gentili, A., & Mulligan, T. (1998). Sexual dysfunction in older adults. *Clinics in Geriatric Medicine, 14,* 383–393.

Glatt, A. E., Zinner, S. H., & McCormack, W. M. (1990). The prevalence of dyspareunia. *Obstetrics and Gynecology, 75,* 433–436.

Goggin, K., Engelson, E. S., Rabkin, J. G., & Kotler, D. P. (1998). The relationship of mood, endocrine, and sexual disorders in human immunodeficiency virus positive (HIV+) women: An exploratory study. *Psychosomatic Medicine, 60,* 11–16.

Golding, J. M. (1996). Sexual assault history and women's reproductive and sexual health. *Psychology of Women Quarterly, 20,* 101–121.

Goldmeier, D., Keane, F. E., Carter, P., Hessman, A., Harris, J. R., & Renton, A.

(1997). Prevalence of sexual dysfunction in heterosexual patients attending a central London genitourinary medicine clinic. *International Journal of STD and AIDS, 8,* 303–306.

Goldstein, I. (1999, October 22–24). *New perspectives in the management of female sexual dysfunction.* Conference, Boston.

Goldstein, J., & Berman, J. (1998). Vasculogenic female sexual dysfunction: Vaginal engorgement and clitoral erectile insufficiency syndromes. *International Journal of Impotence Research, 10,* 584–590.

Gordon, C. M., & Carey, M. P. (1993). Penile tumescence monitoring during morning naps: A pilot investigation of a cost-effective alternative to full night sleep studies in the assessment of male erectile disorder. *Behaviour Research and Therapy, 31,* 503–506.

Gordon, C. M., & Carey, M. P. (1995). Penile tumescence monitoring during morning naps to assess male erectile functioning: An initial study of healthy men of varied ages. *Archives of Sexual Behavior, 24,* 291–307.

Gottman, J., Notarius, C., Gonso, J., & Markman, H. (1976). *A couples guide to communication.* Champaign, IL: Research Press.

Greenwald, E., Leitenberg, H., Cado, S., & Tarran, M. J. (1990). Childhood sexual abuse: Long-term effects on psychological and sexual functioning in a nonclinical and nonstudent sample of adult women. *Child Abuse and Neglect, 14,* 503–513.

Grimes, J. B., & Labbate, L. A. (1996). Spontaneous orgasm with the combined use of bupropion and sertraline. *Biological Psychiatry, 40,* 1184–1185.

Haspel, K. C., Jorgenson, L. M., Wincze, J. P., & Parsons, J. P. (1997). Lesiglative intervention regarding therapist sexual misconduct: An overview. *Professional Psychology: Research and Practice, 28,* 63–72.

Hathaway, S. R., & McKinley, J. C. (1967). *The Minnesota Multiphasic Personality Inventory manual.* New York: Psychological Corporation.

Hatzinger, M., Seemann, O., Grenacher, L., & Rassweiler, J. (1997). Laparoscopy-assisted penile revascularization: A new method. *Journal of Endourology, 4,* 269–272.

Hawatmeh, I., Houttuin, E., Gregory, J., & Purcell, M. (1983). Vascular surgery for the treatment of the impotent male. In R. J. Krane, M. B. Siroky, & I. Goldstein (Eds.), *Male sexual dysfunction* (pp. 291–299). Boston: Little, Brown.

Hawton, K. (1982). The behavioural treatment of sexual dysfunction. *British Journal of Psychiatry, 140,* 94–101.

Hawton, K. (1985). *Sex therapy: A practical guide.* Northvale, NJ: Aronson.

Hawton, K., Catalan, J., & Fagg, J. (1992). Sex therapy for erectile dysfunction: Characteristics of couples, treatment outcome, and prognostic factors. *Archives of Sexual Behavior, 21,* 161–175.

Hawton, K., Gath, D., & Day, A. (1994). Sexual function in a community sample of middle-aged women with partners: Effects of age, marital, socioeconomic, psychiatric, gynecological, and menopausal factors. *Archives of Sexual Behavior, 23,* 375–395.

Heim, N. (1981). Sexual behavior of castrated sex offenders. *Archives of Sexual Behavior, 10,* 11–19.

Heiman, J. R. (2000). Orgasmic disorders in women. In S. R. Leiblum & R. C. Rosen (Eds.), *Principles and practice of sex therapy* (3rd ed., pp. 118–153). New York: Guilford.

Heiman, J. R., & LoPiccolo, J. (1988). *Becoming orgasmic: A sexual and personal growth program for women* (rev. ed.). New York: Prentice-Hall.

Heiman, J. R., & Meston, C. M. (1997). Empirically validated treatment for sexual dysfunction. *Annual Review of Sex Research, 8,* 148–195.

Heisterberg, L. (1993). Factors influencing spontaneous abortion, dyspareunia, dysmenorrhea, and pelvic pain. *Obstetrics and Gynecology, 81,* 594–597.

Herbert, S. E. (1996). Lesbian sexuality. In R. P. Cabaj & T. S. Stein (Eds.), *Textbook of homosexuality and mental health* (pp. 723–742). Washington, DC: American Psychiatric Press.

Herer, E., & Holzapfel, S. (1993). The medical causes of infertility and their effects on sexuality. *Canadian Journal of Human Sexuality, 2,* 113–120.

Hirst, J. F., Baggaley, M. R., & Watson, J. P. (1996). A four-year survey of an inner-city psychosexual problem clinic. *Journal of Sex and Marital Therapy, 11,* 19–36.

Hite, S. (1976). *The Hite report: A nationwide study of female sexuality.* New York: Dell.

Holroyd, J. C., & Brodsky, A. M. (1977). Psychologists' attitudes and practices regarding erotic and nonerotic physical contact with patients. *American Psychologist, 32,* 843–849.

Hong, L. K. (1984). Survival of the fastest: On the origin of premature ejaculation. *Journal of Sex Research, 20,* 109–122.

Hoon, P. W., Wincze, J. P., & Hoon, E. F. (1977). A test of reciprocal inhibition: Are anxiety and sexual arousal in women mutually inhibitory? *Journal of Abnormal Psychology, 86,* 65–74.

Hulter, B. (1999). Sexual function in women with neurological disorders. *Comprehensive Summaries of Uppsala Dissertations from the Faculty of Medicine, 873.* Uppsala, Sweden: Acta Universitatis Upsaliensis.

Hunt, M. (1974). *Sexual behavior in the 70's.* Chicago: Playboy.

Jamieson, D. J., & Steege, J. F. (1996). The prevalence of dysmenorrhea, dyspareunia, pelvic pain, and irritable bowel syndrome in primary care practices. *Obstetrics and Gynecology, 87,* 55–58.

Jarow, J.P., & DeFranzo, A.J. (1996). Long-term results of arterial bypass surgery for impotence secondary to segmental vascular disease. *Journal of Urology, 156,* 982–985.

Jensen, B. J., Witcher, D. B., & Upton, L. R. (1987). Readability assessment of questionnaires frequently used in sex and marital therapy. *Journal of Sex and Marital Therapy, 13,* 137–141.

Jensen, S. B. (1984). Sexual function and dysfunction in younger married alcoholics. *Acta Psychiatrica Scandinavica, 69,* 543–549.

Jetvich, M. J. (1980). Importance of penile arterial pulse sound examination in impotence. *Journal of Urology, 124,* 820–824.

Jindal, U. N., & Dhall, G. I. (1990). Psychosexual problems of infertile women in India. *International Journal of Fertility, 35,* 222–225.

Jones, T. M. (1985). Hormonal considerations in the evaluation and treatment of erectile dysfunction. In R. T. Segraves & H. W. Schoenberg (Eds.), *Diagnosis and treatment of erectile disturbances: A guide for the clinician* (pp. 115–158). New York: Plenum.

Jonler, M., Moon, T., Brannan, W., Stone, N. N., Heisey, D., & Bruskewitz, R. C. (1995). The effect of age, ethnicity and geographical location on impotence and quality of life. *British Journal of Urology, 75,* 651–655.

Kafka, M. P. (2000). The paraphilia-related disorders: Nonparaphilic hypersexuality and sexual compulsivity/addiction. In S. R. Leiblum & R. C. Rosen (Eds.), *Principles and practice of sex therapy* (3rd ed., pp. 471–503). New York: Guilford.

Kalichman, S. C. (1998). *Understanding AIDS: Advances in research and treatment* (2nd ed.). Washington, DC: American Psychological Association.

Kaplan, H. S. (1974). *The new sex therapy.* New York: Brunner/Mazel.

Kaplan, H. S. (1979). *Disorders of sexual desire.* New York: Brunner/Mazel.

Kaplan, H. S. (1989). *How to overcome premature ejaculation.* New York: Brunner/ Mazel.

Kaplan, S. J. (1984). The private practice of behavior therapy. *Progress in Behavior Modification, 17,* 201–240.

Kayigil, O., Ahmed, S. I., & Metin, A. (2000). Deep dorsal vein arterialization in pure cavernoocclusive dysfunction. *European Urology, 37,* 345–349.

Keane, F. E. A., Young, S. M., & Boyle, H. M. (1996). The prevalence of previous sexual assault among routine female attenders at a department of genitourinary medicine. *International Journal of STD and AIDS, 7,* 480–484.

Kelly, J. A. (1995). *Changing HIV risk behavior: Practical strategies.* New York: Guilford.

Kennedy, S. H., Dickens, S. E., Eisfeld, B. S., & Bagby, R. M. (1999). Sexual dysfunction before antidepressant therapy in major depression. *Journal of Affective Disorders, 56,* 201–208.

Kennedy, S. H., Eisfeld, B. S., Dickens, S. E., Bacchiochi, J. R., & Bagby, R. M. (2000). Antidepressant-induced sexual dysfunction during treatment with moclobemide, paroxetine, sertraline, and venlafaxine. *Journal of Clinical Psychiatry, 61,* 276–281.

Kilmann, P. R., Mills, K. H., Caid, C., Bella, B., Davidson, E., & Wanlass, R. (1984). The sexual interaction of women with secondary orgasmic dysfunction and their partners. *Archives of Sexual Behavior, 13,* 41–49.

Kim, E., & Lipshultz, L. (1997). Advances in the treatment of organic erectile dysfunction. *Hospital Practice, 32,* 101–104.

Kinsey, A. C., Pomeroy, W. B., & Martin, C. E. (1948). *Sexual behavior in the human male.* Philadelphia: Saunders.

Kinsey, A. C., Pomeroy, W. B., Martin, C. E., & Gebhard, P. H. (1953). *Sexual behavior in the human female.* Philadelphia: Saunders.

Kinzl, J. F., Traweger, C., & Biebl, W. (1995). Sexual dysfunctions: Relationship to childhood sexual abuse and early family experiences in a nonclinical sample. *Child Abuse and Neglect, 19,* 785–792.

Klassen, A. D., & Wilsnack, S. C. (1986). Sexual experiences and drinking among women in a U.S. national survey. *Archives of Sexual Behavior, 15,* 363–392.

Knapp, S., & VandeCreek, L. (1990). Application of the duty to protect to HIV-positive patients. *Professional Psychology: Research and Practice, 21,* 161–166.

Kolodny, R. C. (1971). Sexual dysfunction in diabetic females. *Diabetes, 20,* 557–559.

Krauss, D. J., Lantinga, L. J., Carey, M. P., Meisler, A. W., & Kelly, C. M. (1989). Use of the malleable penile prosthesis in the treatment of erectile dysfunction: A prospective study of postoperative adjustment. *Journal of Urology, 142,* 988–991.

Laan, E. (1994). *Determinants of sexual arousal in women: Genital and subjective components of sexual response.* Doctoral dissertation, Universitet van Amsterdam, Amsterdam, Netherlands.

Labbate, L. A., Grimes, J. B., & Arana, G. W. (1998). Serotonin reuptake antidepressant effects on sexual function in patients with anxiety disorders. *Biological Psychiatry, 43,* 904–907.

Lamont, J. A. (1978). Vaginismus. *American Journal of Obstetrics and Gynecology, 131,* 632–636.

Langevin, R., Ben-Aron, M. H., Coutland, R., Hucker, S. J., Purins, J. E., Russon, A. E., Day, D., Roper, V., & Webster, C. D. (1985). The effect of alcohol on penile erection. In R. Langevin (Ed.), *Erotic preference, gender identity, and aggression in men: New research studies* (pp. 101–111). Hillsdale, NJ: Erlbaum.

Laumann, E.O., Gagnon, J.H., Michael, R.T., & Michaels, S. (1994). *The social organization of sexuality: Sexual practices in the United States.* Chicago: University of Chicago.

Laumann, E. O., Paik, A., & Rosen, R. C. (1999). Sexual dysfunction in the United States. *Journal of the American Medical Association, 281,* 537–544.

Laws, D. R. (Ed.). (1989). *Relapse prevention with sex offenders.* New York: Guilford.

Laws, D. R., & O'Donohue, W. (Eds.). (1997). *Sexual deviance: Theory, assessment, and treatment.* New York: Guilford.

Lazarus, A. A. (1988). A multimodal perspective on problems of sexual desire. In S. R. Leiblum & R. C. Rosen (Eds.), *Sexual desire disorders* (pp. 145–167). New York: Guilford.

Leiblum, S. R. (2000). Vaginismus: A most perplexing problem. In S. R. Leiblum & R. C. Rosen (Eds.), *Principles and practice of sex therapy* (3rd ed., pp. 154–180). New York: Guilford.

Leland, J. (2000, May 29). The science of women and sex. *Newsweek,* pp. 46–55.

Letourneau, E. J., Resnick, H. S., Kilpatrick, D. G., Saunders, B. E., & Best, C. L. (1996). Comorbidity of sexual problems and posttraumatic stress disorder in female crime victims. *Behavior Therapy, 27,* 321–336.

Levine, G. N. (1996). *Pocket guide to commonly prescribed drugs* (2nd ed.). Stamford, CT: Appleton & Lange.

Levine, S. B., & Yost, M. A. (1976). Frequency of sexual dysfunction in a general gynecological clinic: An epidemiological approach. *Archives of Sexual Behavior, 5,* 229–238.

Lewis, R. W. (1988). Venous surgery for impotence. *Urologic Clinics of North America, 15,* 115–121.

Libman, E., Fichten, C. S., Creti, L., Weinstein, N., Amsel, R., & Brender, W. (1989).

Sleeping and waking-state measurement of erectile function in an aging male population. *Psychological Assessment, 1,* 284–291.

Lief, H. I. (1977). Inhibited sexual desire. *Medical Aspects of Human Sexuality, 7,* 94–95.

Lindal, E., & Stefansson, J. G. (1993). The lifetime prevalence of psychosexual dysfunction among 55 to 57-year-olds in Iceland. *Social Psychiatry and Psychiatric Epidemiology, 28,* 91–95.

Linet, O. I., & Neff, L. L. (1994). Intracavernous prostaglandin E1 in erectile dysfunction. *Clinical Investigator, 72,* 139–149.

Lipsius, S. H. (1987). Prescribing sensate focus without proscribing intercourse. *Journal of Sex and Marital Therapy, 11,* 185–191.

LoPiccolo, J., & Friedman, J. M. (1988). Broad-spectrum treatment of low sexual desire: Integration of cognitive, behavioral, and systemic therapy. In S. R. Leiblum & R. C. Rosen (Eds.), *Sexual desire disorders* (pp. 107–144). New York: Guilford.

LoPiccolo, J., & Heiman, J. R. (1978). Sexual assessment and history interview. In J. LoPiccolo & L. LoPiccolo (Eds.), *Handbook of sex therapy* (pp. 103–112). New York: Plenum.

LoPiccolo, J., & Lobitz, W. C. (1972). The role of masturbation in the treatment of orgasmic dysfunction. *Archives of Sexual Behavior, 2,* 163–171.

LoPiccolo, J., & Stock, W. E. (1986). Treatment of sexual dysfunction. *Journal of Consulting and Clinical Psychology, 54,* 158–167.

Mahmoud, K. Z., el Dakhli, M. R., Fahmi, I. M., & Abdel-Aziz, A. B. (1992). Comparative value of prostaglandin E1 and papaverine in treatment of erectile failure: Double-blind crossover study among Egyptian patients. *Journal of Urology, 147,* 623–626.

Malatesta, V. J., & Adams, H. E. (1984). The sexual dysfunctions. In H. E. Adams & P. B. Sutker (Eds.), *Comprehensive handbook of psychopathology* (pp. 725–775). New York: Plenum.

Malatesta, V. J., Pollack, R. H., Crotty, T. D., & Peacock, L. J. (1982). Acute alcohol intoxication and female orgasmic response. *Journal of Sex Research, 18,* 1–17.

Mannino, D. M., Klevens, R. M., & Flanders, W. D. (1994). Cigarette smoking: An independent risk factor for impotence? *American Journal of Epidemiology, 140,* 1003–1008.

Margolese, H., & Assalian, P. (1996). Sexual side effects of antidepressants: A review. *Journal of Sex and Marital Therapy, 22,* 209–217.

Masters, W. H., & Johnson, V. E. (1966). *Human sexual response.* Boston: Little, Brown.

Masters, W. H., & Johnson, V. E. (1970). *Human sexual inadequacy.* Boston: Little, Brown.

Masters, W. H., Johnson, V. E., & Kolodny, R. C. (1988). *Human sexuality* (3rd ed.). Boston: Little, Brown.

McCabe, M. P., & Cobain, M. J. (1998). The impact of individual and relationship factors on sexual dysfunction among males and females. *Sexual and Marital Therapy, 13,* 131–143.

McCarthy, B. W. (1985). Uses and misuses of behavioral homework exercises in sex therapy. *Journal of Sex and Marital Therapy, 11,* 185–191.

McCarthy, B. W. (1992). Treatment of erectile dysfunction with single men. In R. C. Rosen & S. R. Leiblum (Eds.), *Erectile disorders: Assessment and treatment* (pp. 313–340). New York: Guilford.

McCarthy, B. (1998). *Male sexual awareness: Increasing sexual satisfaction* (rev. and updated ed.). New York: Carroll & Graf.

McCormack W. M., & Spence, M. R. (1999). Evaluation of the surgical treatment of vulvar vestibulitis. *European Journal of Obstetrics, Gynecology, and Reproductive Biology, 86*, 135–138.

McDowell, I., & Newell, C. (1996). *Measuring health: A guide to rating scales and questionnaires.* New York: Oxford University Press.

McGovern, K. B., Stewart, R. C., & LoPiccolo, J. (1975). Secondary orgasmic dysfunction: I. Analysis and strategies for treatment. *Archives of Sexual Behavior, 4*, 265–275.

Meana, M., & Binik Y. M. (1994). Painful coitus: A review of female dyspareunia. *Journal of Nervous and Mental Disease, 182*, 264–272.

Meana, M., Binik, Y. M., Khalifé, S., Bergeron, S., Pagidas, K., & Berkley, K. J. (1997a). Dyspareunia: More than bad sex. *Pain, 71*, 211–212.

Meana, M., Binik, Y. M., Khalifé, S., & Cohen, D. (1997b). Dyspareunia: Sexual dysfunction or pain syndrome? *Journal of Nervous and Mental Disease, 185*, 561–569.

Meana, M., Binik, Y. M., Khalifé, S., & Cohen, D. (1999). Psychosocial correlates of pain attributions in women with dyspareunia. *Psychosomatics, 40*, 497–502.

Meichenbaum, D. H. (1977). *Cognitive-behavior modification: An integrative approach.* New York: Plenum.

Meisler, A. W., & Carey, M. P. (1990). A critical reevaluation of nocturnal penile tumescence monitoring in the diagnosis of erectile dysfunction. *Journal of Nervous and Mental Disease, 178*, 78–89.

Meisler, A. W., & Carey, M. P. (1991). Depressed affect and male sexual arousal. *Archives of Sexual Behavior, 20*, 541–554.

Meisler, A. W., Carey, M. P., Krauss, D. J., & Lantinga, L. J. (1988). Success and failure in penile prosthesis surgery: Two cases highlighting the importance of psychosocial factors. *Journal of Sex and Marital Therapy, 14*, 108–119.

Melchert, T. P., & Patterson, M. M. (1999). Duty to warn and intervention with HIV-positive clients. *Professional Psychology: Research and Practice, 30*, 180–186.

Mendoza, M., & Silverman, M. (1987). Penile prosthetics: Characteristics of veteran patients and their spouses. *Journal of Sex and Marital Therapy, 13*, 183–192.

Meston, C. M., & Gorzalka, B. (1992). Psychoactive drugs and human sexual behavior: The role of serotonergic activity. *Journal of Psychoactive Drugs, 24*, 1–40.

Meston, C. M., & Gorzalka, B. B. (1996). Differential effects of sympathetic activation on sexual arousal in sexually dysfunctional and functional women. *Journal of Abnormal Psychology, 105*, 582–591.

Meston, C. M., Gorzalka, B. B., & Wright, J. (1997). Inhibition of subjective and physiological sexual arousal in women by clonidine. *Psychosomatic Medicine, 59*, 399–407.

Meston, C. M., & Heiman, J. R. (1998). Ephedrine-activated physiological sexual arousal in women. *Archives of General Psychiatry, 55*, 652–656.

Metz, M. E., Pryor, J. L., Nesvacil, L. J., Abuzzahab, F., Sr., & Koznar, J. (1997). Premature ejaculation: A psychophysiological review. *Journal of Sex and Marital Therapy, 23,* 3–23.

Metz, M. E., & Seifert, M. H. (1990). Men's expectations of physicians in sexual health concerns. *Journal of Sex and Marital Therapy, 16,* 79–88.

Meyer-Bahlburg, H. F., Noestlinger, C., Exner, T. M., Ehrhardt, A. A., Gruen, R. S., Lorenz, G., Gorman, J. M., El-Sadr, W., & Sorrell, S. L. (1993). Sexual functioning in HIV+ and HIV– injected drug-using women. *Journal of Sex and Marital Therapy, 19,* 56–68.

Modebe, O. (1990). Erectile failure among medical clinic patients. *African Journal of Medicine and Medical Science, 19,* 259–264.

Moody, G. A., & Mayberry, J. F. (1993). Perceived sexual dysfunction amongst patients with inflammatory bowel disease. *Digestion, 54,* 256–260.

Morganstern, K. P. (1988). Behavioral interviewing. In A. S. Bellack & M. Hersen (Eds.), *Behavioral assessment: A practical handbook* (pp. 86–118). Elmsford, NY: Pergamon Press.

Morokoff, P. J. (1978). Determinants of female orgasm. In J. LoPiccolo & L. LoPiccolo (Eds.), *Handbook of sex therapy* (pp. 147–165). New York: Plenum.

Morokoff, P. J., Baum, A., McKinnon, W. R., & Gillilland, R. (1987). Effects of chronic unemployment and acute psychological stress on sexual arousal in men. *Health Psychology, 6,* 545–560.

Morokoff, P. J., & Heiman, J. R. (1980). Effects of erotic stimuli on sexually functional and dysfunctional women: Multiple measures before and after sex therapy. *Behaviour Research and Therapy, 18,* 127–137.

Morrissette, D., Skinner, M., Hoffmann, B., Levine, R., & Davidson, J. (1993). Effects of antihypertensive drugs atenolol and nifedipine on sexual function in older men: A placebo controlled cross-over study. *Archives of Sexual Behavior, 22,* 99–109.

Moses, J. M., Hord, D. J., Lubin, A., Johnson, L. C., & Naitoh, C. (1975). Dynamics of nap sleep during a 40 hour period. *Electroencephalography and Clinical Neurophysiology, 39,* 627–633.

Moss, H. B., & Procci, W. R. (1982). Sexual dysfunction associated with oral antihypertensive medication: A critical survey of the literature. *General Hospital Psychiatry, 4,* 121–129.

Mullen, P. E., Martin, J. L., Anderson, J. C., Romans, S. E., & Herbison, G. P. (1994). The effect of child sexual abuse on social, interpersonal and sexual function in adult life. *British Journal of Psychiatry, 165,* 35–47.

Munjack, D. J., & Kanno, P. H. (1979). Retarded ejaculation: A review. *Archives of Sexual Behavior, 8,* 139–150.

Nadig, P., Ware, J., & Blumoff, R. (1986). Noninvasive device to produce and maintain an erection-like state. *Urology, 27,* 126–131.

Nettelbladt, P., & Uddenberg, N. (1979). Sexual dysfunction and sexual satisfaction in 58 married Swedish men. *Journal of Psychosomatic Medicine, 23,* 141–147.

Ng, M.-L. (1999). Vaginismus: A disease, symptom or culture-bound syndrome? *Sexual and Marital Therapy, 14,* 9–13.

Nirenberg, T., Wincze, J., Bansal, S., Liepman, M., Engle-Friedman, M., & Begin, A. (1991). Volunteer bias in a study of male alcoholics sexual behavior. *Archives of Sexual Behavior, 20,* 371–380.

Norris, J., & Feldman-Summers, S. (1981). Factors related to the psychological impacts of rape on the victim. *Journal of Abnormal Psychology, 90,* 562–567.

Norton, R., Feldman, C., & Tafoya, D. (1974). Risk parameters across types of secrets. *Journal of Counseling Psychology, 21,* 450–454.

Nunns, D., & Mandal, D. (1997). Psychological and psychosexual aspects of vulvar vestibulitis. *Genitourinary Medicine, 73,* 541–544.

Nurnberg, H. G., Hensley, P. L., Lauriello, J., Parker, L. M., & Keith, S. J. (1999). Sildenafil for women patients with antidepressant-induced sexual dysfunction. *Psychiatric Services, 50,* 1076–1078.

Nusbaum, M. R., Gamble, G., Skinner, B., & Heiman, J. (2000). The high prevalence of sexual concerns among women seeking routine gynecological care. *Journal of Family Practice, 49,* 229–232.

O'Farrell, T. J. (1990). Sexual functioning of male alcoholics. In R. L. Collins, K. E. Leonard, B. A. Miller, & J. S. Searles (Eds.), *Alcohol and the family: research and clinical perspectives* (pp. 244–271). New York: Guilford.

O'Leary, M., & Rosen, R. C. (1997, May). Paper presented at the Cape Cod Conference on Assessment of Sexual Function in Clinical Trials: Male Sexuality, Hyannis, MA.

O'Leary, M., & Rosen, R. C. (1998, May). Paper presented at the Cape Cod Conference on Assessment of Sexual Function in Clinical Trials: Female Sexuality, Hyannis, MA.

O'Sullivan, K. (1979). Observation on vaginismus in Irish women. *Archives of General Psychiatry, 36,* 824–826.

Pace, J., Brown, G. R., Rundell, J. R., & Paolucci, S. (1990). Prevalence of psychiatric disorders in a mandatory screening program for infection with human immunodeficiency virus: A pilot study. *Military Medicine, 155,* 76–80.

Palace, E. M. (1995a). Modification of dysfunctional patterns of sexual response through automatic arousal and false physiological feedback [Correction]. *Journal of Consulting and Clinical Psychology, 63,* 809.

Palace, E. M. (1995b). Modification of dysfunctional patterns of sexual response through autonomic arousal and false physiological feedback. *Journal of Consulting and Clinical Psychology, 63,* 604–615.

Palace, E. M., & Gorzalka, B. B. (1990). The enhancing effects of anxiety on arousal in sexually dysfunctional and functional women. *Journal of Abnormal Psychology, 99,* 403–411.

Panser, L., Rhodes, T., Girman, C., Guess, H., Chute, C., Oesterling, J., Lieber, M., & Jacobsen, S. (1995). Sexual function of men ages 40 to 79 years: The Olmsted County Study of Urinary Symptoms and Health Status among Men. *Journal of American Geriatric Society, 43,* 1107–1111.

Papadopoulos, C. (1989). *Sexual aspects of cardiovascular disease.* New York: Praeger.

Parshley, H. M. (1933). Sexual abstinence as a biological question. *Scientific American, 148,* 283–300.

Pedersen, B., & Mohl, B. (1991). Behind every penis is a man. *Nordisk-Sexological, 9,* 226–231.

Pedersen, B., Tiefer, L., Ruiz, M., & Melman, A. (1988). Evaluation of patients and partners 1 to 4 years after penile prosthesis surgery. *Journal of Urology, 139,* 956–958.

Poinsard, P. J. (1966). Psychophysiologic (psychosomatic) disorders of the vulvovaginal tract. *Psychosomatics, 7,* 338–342.

Pope, B. (1979). *The mental health interview: Research and application.* Elmsford, NY: Pergamon.

Purnine, D. M., & Carey, M. P. (1997). Interpersonal communication and sexual adjustment: The role of understanding and agreement. *Journal of Consulting and Clinical Psychology, 65,* 1017–1025.

Purnine, D. M., & Carey, M. P. (1998). Age and gender differences in sexual behavior preferences: A follow-up report. *Journal of Sex and Marital Therapy, 24,* 27–36.

Purnine, D. M., & Carey, M. P. (1999). Dyadic coorientation: Re-examination of a method for studying interpersonal communication. *Archives of Sexual Behavior, 28,* 45–62.

Purnine, D. M., Carey, M. P., & Jorgensen, R. S. (1996). The Inventory of Dyadic Heterosexual Preferences (IDHP): Development and psychometric evaluation of a measure of couples' preferred sexual scripts. *Behaviour Research and Therapy, 34,* 375–387.

Rakic, Z., Starcevic, V., Starcevic, V. P., & Marinkovic, J. (1997). Testosterone treatment in men with erectile disorder and low testosterone in serum. *Archives of Sexual Behavior, 26,* 495–504.

Read, S., King, M., & Watson, J. (1997). Sexual dysfunction in primary medical care: Prevalence, characteristics and detection by the general practitioner. *Journal of Public Health Medicine, 19,* 387–391.

Reamy, K. J., & White, S. E. (1985). Dyspareunia in pregnancy. *Journal of Psychosomatic Obstetrics and Gynaecology, 4,* 263–270.

Reissing, E. D., Binik, Y. M., & Khalifé, S. (1999). Does vaginismus exist? A critical review of the literature. *Journal of Nervous and Mental Disease, 187,* 261–274.

Rekers, H., Drogendijk, A. C., Valkenburg, H. A., & Riphagen, F. (1992). The menopause, urinary incontinence and other symptoms of the genitourinary tract. *Maturitas, 15,* 101–111.

Renshaw, D. C. (1988). Profile of 2,376 patients treated at Loyola Sex Clinic between 1972 and 1987. *Sexual and Marital Therapy, 3,* 111–117.

Roehrich, L., & Kinder, B. (1991). Alcohol expectancies and male sexuality: Review and implications for sex therapy. *Journal of Sex and Marital Therapy, 17,* 45–54.

Rosen, R. C., & Beck, J. G. (1988). *Patterns of sexual arousal: Psychophysiological processes and clinical applications.* New York: Guilford.

Rosen, R. C., Kostis, J. B., & Jekelis, A. W. (1988). Beta-blocker effects on sexual function in normal males. *Archives of Sexual Behavior, 17,* 241–255.

Rosen, R. C., Kostis, J. B., Jekelis, A. W., & Taska, L. (1994). Sexual sequelae of antihypertensive drugs: Treatment effects on self-report and physiological measures in middle-aged male hypertensives. *Archives of Sexual Behavior, 23,* 135–152.

Rosen, R. C., & Leiblum, S. R. (Eds.). (1992). *Erectile disorders: Assessment and treatment.* New York: Guilford.

Rosen, R. C., Leiblum, S. R., & Spector, I. P. (1994). Psychologically based treatment for male erectile disorder: A cognitive-interpersonal model. *Journal of Sex and Marital Therapy, 20,* 67–85.

Rosen, R. C., Riley, A., Wagner, G., Osterloh, I. H., Kirkpatrick, J., & Mishra, A. (1997). The International Index of Erectile Function (IIEF): A multidimensional scale for assessment of erectile dysfunction. *Urology, 49,* 822–830.

Rosen, R. C., Taylor, J., Leiblum, S. R., & Bachmann, G. (1993). Prevalence of sexual dysfunction in women: Results of a survey study in 329 women in an outpatient gynecological clinic. *Journal of Sex and Marital Therapy, 19,* 171–188.

Rosser, B. R., Metz, M. E., Bockting, W. O., & Buroker, T. (1997). Sexual difficulties, concerns, and satisfaction in homosexual men: An empirical study with implications for HIV prevention. *Journal of Sex and Marital Therapy, 23,* 61–73.

Rossman, B., Mieza, M., & Melman, A. (1990). Penile vein ligation for corporeal incompetence: An evaluation of short-term and long-term results. *Journal of Urology, 144,* 679–682.

Rous, S. N. (1988). *The prostate book: Sound advice on symptoms and treatment.* Mount Vernon, NY: Consumers Union.

Rowland, D., Cooper, S., Slob, A., Koos, A., & Houtsmuller, E. (1997). The study of ejaculatory response in men in the psychophysiological Laboratory. *Journal of Sex Research, 34,* 161–166.

Ruzbarsky, V., & Michal, V. (1977). Morphologic changes in the arterial bed of the penis with aging: Relationship to the pathogenesis of impotence. *Investigative Urology, 15,* 194–199.

Sakheim, D., Barlow, D. H., Abrahamson, D. J., & Beck, J. G. (1987). Distinguishing between organogenic and psychogenic erectile dysfunction. *Behaviour Research and Therapy, 25,* 379–390.

Sakheim, D., Barlow, D. H., Beck, J. G., & Abrahamson, D. (1984). The effect of an increased awareness of erectile cues on sexual arousal. *Behaviour Research and Therapy, 22,* 151–158.

Salerian, A. J., Deibler, W. E., Vittone, B. J., Geyer, S. P., Drell, L., Mirmirani, N., Mirczak, J. A., Byrd, W., Tunick, S. B., Wax, M., & Fleisher, S. (2000). Sildenafil for psychotropic-induced sexual dysfunction in 31 women and 61 men. *Journal of Sex and Marital Therapy, 26,* 133–140.

Salmimies, P., Kockott, G., Pirke, K. M., Vogt, H. J., & Schill, W. B. (1982). Effects of testosterone replacement on sexual behavior in hypogonadal men. *Archives of Sexual Behavior, 11,* 345–353.

Sarramon, J.P., Bertrand, N., Malavaud, B., & Rischmann, P. (1997). Microrevascularization of the penis in vascular impotence. *International Journal of Impotence Research, 9,* 127–133.

Sarrel, P. M. (2000). Effects of hormone replacement therapy on sexual psychophysiology and behavior in postmenopause. *Journal of Women's Health and Gender Based Medicine, 9*(Suppl. 1), S-32.

Sarwer, D. B., & Durlak, J. A. (1996). Childhood sexual abuse as a predictor of adult female sexual dysfunction: A study of couples seeking sex therapy. *Child Abuse and Neglect, 20,* 963–972.

Sarwer, D. B., & Durlak, J. A. (1997). A field trial of the effectiveness of behavioral treatment for sexual dysfunctions. *Journal of Sex and Marital Therapy, 23,* 87–97.

Sasso, F., Gulino, G., Di-Pinto, A., & Alcini, E. (1996). Should venous surgery still be proposed or neglected? *International Journal of Impotency Research, 8,* 25–28.

Schiavi, R. C., Mandeli, J., Schreiner-Engel, P., & Chambers, A. (1991). Aging, sleep disorders, and male sexual function. *Biological Psychiatry, 30,* 15–24.

Schiavi, R. C., Stimmel, B. B., Mandeli, J., & White, D. (1995). Chronic alcoholism and male sexual function. *American Journal of Psychiatry, 152,* 1045–1051.

Schiavi, R. C., White, D., Mandeli, J., & Levine, A. (1997). Effects of testosterone administration on sexual behavior and mood in men with erectile dysfunction. *Archives of Sexual Behavior, 26,* 231–241.

Schoener, G. R., Milgrom, J. H., Gonsiorek, J. C., Luepker, E. T., & Conroe, R. M. (Eds.). (1990). *Psychotherapists' sexual involvement with clients: Intervention and prevention.* Minneapolis, MN: Walk-In Counseling Center.

Schover, L. R. (1989). Sex therapy for the penile prosthesis recipient. *Urologic Clinics of North America, 16,* 91–98.

Schover, L. R., Friedman, J. M., Weiler, S. J., Heiman, J. R., & LoPiccolo, J. (1982). Multiaxial problem-oriented system for sexual dysfunctions: An alternative to DSM-III. *Archives of General Psychiatry, 39,* 614–619.

Schover, L. R., & Jensen, S. B. (1988). *Sexuality and chronic illness: A comprehensive approach.* New York: Guilford.

Schreiner-Engel, P., Schiavi, R. C., Vietorisz, D., Eichel, J. D., & Smith, H. (1985). Diabetes and female sexuality: A comparative study of women in relationships. *Journal of Sex and Marital Therapy, 11,* 165–175.

Scott, F., Bradley, W., & Timm, G. (1973). Management of erectile impotence: Use of implantable inflatable prosthesis. *Urology, 2,* 80–82.

Segraves, K., & Segraves, R.T. (1991). Hypoactive sexual desire disorder: Prevalence and comorbidity in 906 subjects. *Journal of Sex and Marital Therapy, 17,* 55–58.

Segraves, R. T. (1988). Drugs and desire. In S. R. Leiblum & R. C. Rosen (Eds.), *Sexual desire disorders* (pp. 313–347). New York: Guilford Press.

Segraves, R. T. (1995). Antidepressant-induced orgasm disorder. *Journal of Sex and Marital Therapy, 21,* 192–201.

Segraves, R. T., Madsen, R., Carter, C. S., & Davis, J. M. (1985). Erectile dysfunction associated with pharmacological agents. In R. T. Segraves & H. W. Schoenberg (Eds.), *Diagnosis and treatment of erectile disturbances: A guide for clinicians* (pp. 23–63). New York: Plenum.

Segraves R. T., Saran, A., Segraves, K., & Maguire, E. (1993). Clomipramine versus placebo in the treatment of premature ejaculation: A pilot study. *Journal of Sex and Marital Therapy, 19,* 198–200.

Seligman, M. E. P. (1975). *Helplessness: On depression, development, and death.* San Francisco: Freeman.

Semans, J. H. (1956). Premature ejaculation: A new approach. *Southern Medical Journal, 49,* 353–358.

Shah, R.S., & Kulkarni, V.R. (1995). Penile revascularization: An overview. *Annals of Academic Medicine of Singapore, 24,* 749–754.

Shahar, E., Lederer, J., & Herz, M. J. (1991). The use of a self-report questionnaire to assess the frequency of sexual dysfunction in family practice clinics. *Family Practice, 8,* 206–212.

Shen, W. W., & Hsu, J. H. (1995). Female sexual side effects associated with selective serotonin reuptake inhibitors: A descriptive clinical study of 33 patients. *International Journal of Psychiatry in Medicine, 25,* 239–248.

Sherwin, B. B. (1985). Changes in sexual behavior as a function of plasma sex steroid levels in post-menopausal women. *Maturitas, 7,* 225–233.

Sherwin, B. B. (1988). A comparative analysis of the role of androgen in human male and female sexual behavior: Behavioral specificity, critical thresholds and sensitivity. *Psychobiology, 16,* 416–425.

Sherwin, B. B., & Gelfand, M. M. (1987). The role of androgen in the maintenance of sexual functioning in oophorectomized women. *Psychosomatic Medicine, 49,* 397–409.

Sherwin, B. B., Gelfand, M. M., & Brender, W. (1985). Androgen enhances sexual motivation in females: A prospective, crossover study of sex steroid administration in the surgical menopause. *Psychosomatic Medicine, 47,* 339–351.

Shires, A., & Miller, D. (1998). A preliminary study comparing psychological factors associated with erectile dysfunction in heterosexual and homosexual men. *Sexual and Marital Therapy, 13,* 37–49.

Shokrollahi, P., Mirmohamadi, M., Mehrabi, F., & Babaei, G. (1999). Prevalence of sexual dysfunction in women seeking services at family planning centers in Tehran. *Journal of Sex and Marital Therapy, 25,* 211–215.

Shull, G. R., & Sprenkle, D. H. (1980). Retarded ejaculation: Reconceptualization and implications for treatment. *Journal of Sex and Marital Therapy, 6,* 234–246.

Simons, J. S., & Carey, M. P. (2001). Prevalence of the sexual dysfunctions: Results from a decade of research. *Archives of Sexual Behavior, 30,* 177–219.

Singer, C., Weiner, W. J., & Sanchez-Ramos, J. R. (1992). Autonomic dysfunction in men with Parkinson's disease. *European Journal of Neurology, 32,* 134–140.

Small, M. P., Carrion, H. M., & Gordon, J. A. (1975). Small–Carrion penile prosthesis: New implant for management of impotence. *Urology, 5,* 479–486.

Solano, C. H. (1981). Sex differences and the Taylor–Altman self-disclosure stimuli. *Journal of Social Psychology, 115,* 287–288.

Solstad, K., & Hertoft, P. (1993). Frequency of sexual problems and sexual dysfunction in middle-aged Danish men. *Archives of Sexual Behavior, 22,* 51–58.

Spanier, G. B. (1976). Measuring dyadic adjustment: New scales for assessing the quality of marriage and similar dyads. *Journal of Marriage and the Family, 38,* 15–28.

Speckens, A. E. M., Hengeveld, M. W., Nijeholt, G. L., van Hemert, A. M., & Hawton, K. E. (1995). Psychosexual functioning of partners of men with presumed nonorganic erectile dysfunction: Cause or consequence of the disorder? *Archives of Sexual Behavior, 24,* 157–172.

Spector, I. P., & Carey, M. P. (1990). Incidence and prevalence of the sexual dysfunctions: A critical review of the empirical literature. *Archives of Sexual Behavior, 19,* 389–408.

Spector, I. P., Carey, M. P., & Steinberg, L. (1996). The Sexual Desire Inventory: Development, factor structure, and evidence of reliability. *Journal of Sex and Marital Therapy, 22,* 175–190.

Spector, I. P., Leiblum, S. R., Carey, M. P., & Rosen, R. C. (1993). Diabetes and female sexual function: A critical review. *Annals of Behavioral Medicine, 15,* 257–264.

Steege, J. F. (1984). Dyspareunia and vaginismus. *Clinical Obstetrics and Gynecology, 27,* 750–759.

Stoller, R. J. (1975). *Perversion: The erotic form of hatred.* New York: Pantheon Books.

Sundaram, C., Thomas, W., Pryor, L., Sidi, A., Billups, K., & Pryor, J. (1997). Long-term follow-up of patients receiving injection therapy for erectile dysfunction. *Urology, 49,* 932–933.

Szasz, T. (1980). *Sex by prescription.* Garden City, NY: Doubleday/Anchor.

Tan, E. T., Johnson, R. H., Lambie, D. G., Vijayasenan, M. E., & Whiteside, E. A. (1984). Erectile impotence in chronic alcoholics. *Alcoholism: Clinical and Experimental Research, 8,* 297–301.

Taylor, J. F., Rosen, R. C., & Leiblum S. R. (1994). Self-report assessment of female sexual function: Psychometric evaluation of the Brief Index of Sexual Functioning for women. *Archives of Sexual Behavior, 23,* 627–643.

Thompson, A., Lake, K., & Richards, C. (1994). Frequently cited sources in human sexology: A nineties update. *Journal of Sex and Marital Therapy, 20,* 237–243.

Tiefer, L., Pedersen, B., & Melman, A. (1988). Psychosocial follow-up of penile prosthesis implant patients and partner. *Journal of Sex and Marital Therapy, 14,* 184–201.

Tissot, S. A. D. (1766). *On onania: Or a treatise upon the disorders produced by masturbation* (trans. A. Hume). London: Pridden.

Tobias, P. (1975). *Project foundation: An annotated bibliography of scientific studies done since 1900 on sexual abstinence.* Houston, TX: Institute for the Cultural and Scientific Study of Chastity.

Tollison, C. D., & Adams, H. E. (1979). *Sexual disorders: Treatment, theory, and research.* New York: Gardner.

Trudel, G., Boulos, L., & Matte, B. (1993). Dyadic adjustment in couples with hypoactive sexual desire disorders. *Journal of Sex Education and Therapy, 19,* 31–36.

Tsai, M., Feldman-Summers, S., & Edgar, M. (1979). Childhood molestation: Variables related to differential impact on psychosexual functioning in adult women. *Journal of Abnormal Psychology, 88,* 404–414.

Tugrul, C., & Kabakci, E. (1997). Vaginismus and its correlates. *Sexual and Marital Therapy, 12,* 23–34.

Turkat, I. D. (1986). The behavioral interview. In A. R. Ciminero, K. S. Calhoun, & H. E. Adams (Eds.), *Handbook of behavioral assessment* (2nd ed., pp. 109–149). New York: Wiley.

Turner, L. A., & Althof, S. E. (1992). The clinical effectiveness of self-injection and external vacuum devices in the treatment of erectile dysfunction: A six-month comparison. *Psychiatric Medicine, 10,* 283–293.

van Lankveld, J. J. D. M. (1998). Bibliotherapy in the treatment of sexual dysfunctions: A meta-analysis. *Journal of Consulting and Clinical Psychology, 66,* 702–708.

Ventegodt, S. (1998). Sex and the quality of life in Denmark. *Archives of Sexual Behavior, 27,* 295–307.

Verma, K. K., Khaitan, B. K., & Singh, O. P. (1998). The frequency of sexual dysfunctions in patients attending a sex therapy clinic in north India. *Archives of Sexual Behavior, 27,* 309–314.

Viosca, K., & Griner, B. (1988). *Use of the Erec-Aide in the management of impotence.* Paper presented at the meeting of the Endocrine Society, New Orleans, LA.

Virag, R. (1999). Indications and early results of sildenafil (Viagra) in erectile dysfunction. *Urology, 54,* 1073–1077.

Wagner, G., & Metz, P. (1981). Arteriosclerosis and erectile failure. In G. Wagner & R. Green (Eds.), *Impotence: Physiological, psychological, surgical diagnosis and treatment* (pp. 63–72). New York: Plenum.

Walling, M., Andersen, B. L., & Johnson, S. R. (1990). Hormonal replacement therapy for postmenopausal women: A review of sexual outcomes and related gynecologic effects. *Archives of Sexual Behavior, 19,* 119–137.

Wallis, L. A. (1987). Management of dyspareunia in postmenopausal women. *Journal of the American Medical Women's Association, 42,* 82–84.

Wasti, S., Robinson, S. C., Akhtar, Y., Khan, S., & Badaruddin, N. (1993). Characteristics of menopause in three socioeconomic urban groups in Karachi, Pakistan. *Maturitas, 16,* 61–69.

Webb, W. B., Agnew, H. W., Jr., & Sternthal, H. (1966). Sleep during the early morning. *Psychonomic Science, 6,* 277–278.

Weber, A. M., Walters, M. D., Schover, L. R., & Mitchinson, A. (1995). Vaginal anatomy and sexual function. *Obstetrics and Gynecology, 86,* 946–949.

Wei, M., Macera, C. A., Davis, D. R., Hornung, C. A., Nankin, H. R., & Blair, S. N. (1994). Total cholesterol and high density lipoprotein cholesterol as important predictors of erectile dysfunction. *American Journal of Epidemiology, 140,* 930–937.

Weinhardt, L. S., & Carey, M. P. (1996). Prevalence of erectile disorder among men with diabetes mellitus: Review of the empirical literature. *Journal of Sex Research, 33,* 205–214.

Weisberg, R., Brown, T., Wincze, J., & Barlow, D. (2000, June). *Psychological factors and vulnerability to sexual dysfunction: The role of causal attributions.* Paper presented at the 26th Annual Meeting of the International Academy of Sex Research, Paris, France.

Werner, A. (1939). Male climacteric. *Journal of the American Medical Association, 112,* 1441–1443.

White, G., & Jantos, M. (1998). Sexual behavior changes with vulvar vestibulitis syndrome. *Journal of Reproductive Medicine, 43,* 783–789.

Wilsnack, S. C. (1984). Drinking, sexuality, and sexual dysfunction in women. In S. C. Wilsnack & L. J. Beckman (Eds.), *Alcohol problems in women: Antecedents, consequences, and intervention* (pp. 189–227). New York: Guilford Press.

Wilson, G. T. (1981). The effects of alcohol on human sexual behavior. *Advances in Substance Abuse, 2,* 1–40.

Wincze, J. P. (1982). Assessment of sexual disorders. *Behavioral Assessment, 4,* 257–271.

Wincze, J. P. (2000). Assessment and treatment of atypical sexual behavior. In S. R. Leiblum & R. C. Rosen (Eds.), *Principles and practice of sex therapy* (3rd ed., pp. 449–470). New York: Guilford Press.

Wincze, J. P., Bansal, S., Malhotra, C. M., Balko, A., Susset, J. G., & Malamud, M. A. (1988). A comparison of nocturnal penile tumescence and penile response to erotic stimulation during waking states in comprehensively diagnosed groups of males experiencing erectile difficulties. *Archives of Sexual Behavior, 17,* 333–348.

Wincze, J. P., & Barlow, D. H. (1997a). *Enhancing sexuality: A problem solving approach.* San Antonio, TX: Psychological Corp.

Wincze, J. P., & Barlow, D. H. (1997b). *Enhancing sexuality: Client workbook.* San Antonio, TX: Psychological Corp.

Wincze, J. P., & Barlow, D. H. (1997c). *Enhancing sexuality: Therapist guide.* San Antonio, TX: Psychological Corp.

Wiseneberg, S. L. (1996). Big Ruthie imagines sex without pain. In B. Henderson (Ed.), *The Pushcart Prize XXI.* Wainscott, NY: Pushcart.

Witherington, R. (1988). Suction device therapy in the management of erectile impotence. *Urologic Clinics of North America, 15,* 123–128.

Wolchik, S. A., Beggs, V., Wincze, J. P., Sakheim, D. K., Barlow, D. H., & Mavissakalian, M. (1980). The effects of emotional arousal on subsequent sexual arousal in men. *Journal of Abnormal Psychology, 89,* 595–598.

Wouda, J. C., Hartman, P. M., Bakker, R. M., Bakker, J. O., van de Wiel, H. B. M., & Schultz, W. C. M. W. (1998). Vaginal plethysmography in women with dyspareunia. *Journal of Sex Research, 35,* 141–147.

Zeiss, A. M., Davies, H. D., Wood, M., & Tinklenberg, J. R. (1990). The incidence and correlates of erectile problems in patients with Alzheimer's disease. *Archives of Sexual Behavior, 19,* 325–331.

Zilbergeld, B. (1999). *The new male sexuality* (rev. ed.). New York: Bantam.

Zonana, H. (1989). Warning third parties at risk of AIDS: APA's policy is a reasonable approach. *Hospital and Community Psychiatry, 40,* 162–164.

Index